USING MUSIC IN CHILD AND ADOLESCENT PSYCHOTHERAPY

CREATIVE ARTS AND PLAY THERAPY
Cathy A. Malchiodi and David A. Crenshaw,
Series Editors

This series highlights action-oriented therapeutic approaches that utilize art, play, music, dance/movement, drama, and related modalities. Emphasizing current best practices and research, experienced practitioners show how creative arts and play therapies can be integrated into overall treatment for individuals of all ages. Books in the series provide richly illustrated guidelines and techniques for addressing trauma, attachment problems, and other psychological difficulties, as well as for supporting resilience and self-regulation.

Creative Arts and Play Therapy for Attachment Problems
Cathy A. Malchiodi and David A. Crenshaw, Editors

Play Therapy:
A Comprehensive Guide to Theory and Practice
David A. Crenshaw and Anne L. Stewart, Editors

Creative Interventions with Traumatized Children,
Second Edition
Cathy A. Malchiodi, Editor

Music Therapy Handbook
Barbara L. Wheeler, Editor

Play Therapy Interventions to Enhance Resilience
David A. Crenshaw, Robert Brooks, and Sam Goldstein, Editors

What to Do When Children Clam Up in Psychotherapy:
Interventions to Facilitate Communication
Cathy A. Malchiodi and David A. Crenshaw, Editors

Doing Play Therapy:
From Building the Relationship to Facilitating Change
Terry Kottman and Kristin K. Meany-Walen

Using Music in Child and Adolescent Psychotherapy
Laura E. Beer and Jacqueline C. Birnbaum

Using Music in Child and Adolescent Psychotherapy

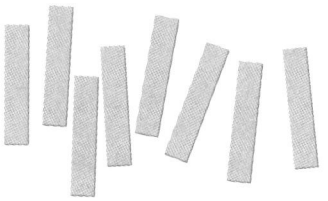

Laura E. Beer
Jacqueline C. Birnbaum

*Series Editors' Note
by Cathy A. Malchiodi and David A. Crenshaw*

THE GUILFORD PRESS
New York   London

Copyright © 2019 The Guilford Press
A Division of Guilford Publications, Inc.
370 Seventh Avenue, Suite 1200, New York, NY 10001
www.guilford.com

All rights reserved

No part of this book may be reproduced, translated, stored in a retrieval system, or transmitted, in any form or by any means, electronic, mechanical, photocopying, microfilming, recording, or otherwise, without written permission from the publisher.

Printed in the United States of America

This book is printed on acid-free paper.

Last digit is print number: 9 8 7 6 5 4 3 2 1

The authors have checked with sources believed to be reliable in their efforts to provide information that is complete and generally in accord with the standards of practice that are accepted at the time of publication. However, in view of the possibility of human error or changes in behavioral, mental health, or medical sciences, neither the authors, nor the editor and publisher, nor any other party who has been involved in the preparation or publication of this work warrants that the information contained herein is in every respect accurate or complete, and they are not responsible for any errors or omissions or the results obtained from the use of such information. Readers are encouraged to confirm the information contained in this book with other sources.

Library of Congress Cataloging-in-Publication Data
Names: Beer, Laura E. | Birnbaum, Jacqueline, C.
Title: Using music in child and adolescent psychotherapy / Laura E. Beer,
    Jacqueline C. Birnbaum.
Description: New York, NY : Guilford Press, [2019] | Series: Creative arts
    and play therapy | Includes bibliographical references and index. |
    Identifiers: LCCN 2018057169 (print) | ISBN 9781462539147 (paperback :
    alk. paper) | ISBN 9781462539154 (hard cover : alk. paper)
Subjects: LCSH: Music therapy. | Child psychotherapy. | Adolescent
    psychotherapy.
Classification: LCC ML3920 (ebook) | LCC ML3920 .B28 2019 (print) | DDC
    615.8/5154—dc23
LC record available at *https://lccn.loc.gov/20180571569*

To all the clients I have had the pleasure of working with, this book is dedicated to you. Your courage, wisdom, and willingness to discover change through music has been my inspiration. I also dedicate this book to my parents, Ed and Rena Beer. They gave me and my siblings (Dave, Peggy, and Bill) a deep appreciation for music and the arts as well as a lifelong love of learning. I am proud to be their daughter. Jackie, this has been such a wonderful collaboration—thank you for an amazing writing experience. And to Cyndy: It seems trite to say I could not have done this without you, but it is true. I really couldn't have. Your love, delicious dinners, and encouragement have brought me this far.

—L. E. B.

Writing this book has been a labor of love—love for music, and all that it can bring to people to improve their lives—as well as an experience of challenge and friendship. I owe a debt of gratitude to Laura for inviting me to go along with her on this adventure; it has been a true pleasure. Thank you, Dean, for your unflagging support as I undertook this project; it meant the world to me. I dedicate this book to my father, Marvin, who passed on to me his love of words and the English language, and to my mother, Flora, paralyzed by polio, who taught me resilience and grace.
I hope they would be proud.

—J. C. B.

About the Authors

Laura E. Beer, PhD, MT-BC, is a board-certified music therapist and Associate Professor and Director of the Music Therapy Program at Maryville University. Since 1988, she has worked in many different settings with children with developmental and psychiatric issues, and with infants in neonatal intensive care units, as well as with older adults and patients in hospice care. Dr. Beer has published on the creative use of music in research and therapy, presented internationally, and facilitated numerous trainings for caregivers for people with advanced dementia. She has received recognition for professional practice and for being a changemaker and advocate for music therapy licensure. Dr. Beer serves as Editor-in-Chief of one of the two national peer-reviewed music therapy journals, *Music Therapy Perspectives*.

Jacqueline C. Birnbaum, MSEd, MA, MT-BC, LCAT, is an early childhood educator, board-certified music therapist, and licensed creative arts therapist. She began her music therapy work in the 1980s in schools for children with communication and other challenges, developing and implementing music therapy programs. Ms. Birnbaum is Administrative Coordinator and Senior Clinician at the Nordoff–Robbins Center for Music Therapy at New York University. She has presented internationally on the use of creative music therapy; is a pianist, guitarist, violinist, composer, and author of published songs for therapy; and is the author of an e-book that includes video examples of her clinical work with a traumatized child. Ms. Birnbaum has served as Chairperson of the Certification Board for Music Therapists.

Series Editors' Note

We all recognize the immediate power of music—how singing a favorite song can make you happy or soothe and calm you, or how listening to a tune can immediately take you back in time to a memory or an important event. Music moves us to tap our feet or clap our hands, or inspires us to get up and dance.

Neuroscientific studies demonstrate just how engagement with music changes our lives in numerous and far-reaching ways. For example, when we sing, neurons in our brains interact in new and different ways and release endorphins and oxytocin (the bonding hormone) that improve mood and quality of life. When we sing together, these effects are amplified: Singing synchronizes our heartbeats and gives us a sense of community. Other studies underscore how listening to music helps to self-regulate mind and body, supports memory retention, and improves cognitive functioning.

Music plays an important role in children's growth and development. Caregivers sing lullabies while rocking infants to sleep, sing songs to teach basic concepts such as the alphabet, or hum tunes during difficult moments and challenges. There is now considerable support for how musical engagement can enhance individual development, attachment, and empathy.

Using Music in Child and Adolescent Psychotherapy is a valuable addition to our series, Creative Arts and Play Therapy, which demonstrates how expressive therapies can be integrated within treatment with children and adolescents. This book and others in the series provide therapists with accessible strategies that complement traditional verbal approaches. When working with children who may not be able to communicate their experiences with words, it is essential that therapists are able to apply creative arts and play-based interventions to effectively assist young clients.

We were delighted to have Laura E. Beer and Jacqueline C. Birnbaum, both experts in the field of music therapy with children and adolescents, write this book, which provides clear guidelines and ideas for therapists who may already be using music or are looking for new ways to reach and work with their child clients. We hope that this volume will enable practitioners to expand their clinical skills and to integrate music into their work with a variety of childhood challenges—trauma, attachment problems, psychosocial issues, and emotional, behavioral, and developmental disorders. The authors skillfully articulate how therapists without any special skills or expertise in music can harness the power of singing, drumming, improvising, or simply listening to music to deepen relationships with their clients and create positive change within the therapeutic milieu.

CATHY A. MALCHIODI, PhD
DAVID A. CRENSHAW, PhD

Preface

> Through music a child enters a world of beauty, expresses his inmost self, tastes the joy of creating, widens his sympathies, develops his mind, soothes and refines his spirit and adds grace to his body.
> —U.S. National Child Welfare Association

Music makes us laugh, cry, and dance, gives us the motivation to complete difficult feats, and helps us feel like we are part of a community. Human culture is saturated with music. If you question this idea, try going through a typical day and listen for how many times music is playing around you. Whether as background music on television or in stores, or as part of your favorite playlist, it is a constant and powerful presence in our lives. Music also has strong therapeutic effects, so clinicians and educators instinctively use music in their work. Let us offer the example of a recent television advertisement. It opens with a man dressed in scrubs talking to a young girl who is lying in a hospital bed. He is kind, warm, and funny, yet she responds tentatively with just a few words and brief eye contact. He begins to sing a name game song and suddenly she looks up at him and immediately joins in the singing. They connect through the song and are smiling at each other. Then he tells her the dreaded shot in the arm is over with and she laughs, saying, "Is it really?" The ad is designed to thank nurses for their work, and it depicts a moment that clearly shows how music is frequently used as a natural part of treatment. The purpose of this book is to help professionals learn how to understand and use music in their clinical practice as a way to access children's inherent strengths and abilities.

A belief in the power of music has sparked much interest in how and why music affects us so deeply. We view music as a universal human trait, as instinctive and natural to life as is breathing. We are all born with the capacity to find meaning in musical experience. All cultures create lullabies; all parents intuitively launch into baby-speak as a way to communicate with, soothe, and connect with their child. Each of us is born hardwired for language and music. Both the language we speak and the music we respond to are shaped by our familial and cultural surroundings. Paul Nordoff and Clive Robbins (1985), pioneers in the field of music therapy, wrote that "music is a universal experience in the sense that all can share in it; its fundamental elements of melody, harmony, and rhythm appeal to, and engage [the] related psychic functions in each of us" (p. 15). This view is supported by the extensive research on the brain being conducted in laboratories and hospitals. Scientists are studying what happens to brain waves and neurological functions when someone is listening to or playing music. Music, unlike speech, motor functions, pain responses, and emotions, is held in every area of the brain. When we listen to a piece of music, our frontal lobes respond to the lyrics, our amygdala responds to the emotional tone, our hippocampus brings up long-held memories related to the song, and our motor neurons make us instinctively move to the beat. Nothing else in the human experience gives us this total response! People who have experienced serious trauma are able to respond to music when words fail them, for music, quite literally, opens up pathways of memories and feelings that are blocked. It is natural that mental health and allied health practitioners will want to find ways to use music to help clients reach their goals.

This book was written to help mental health clinicians, health professionals, and educators understand how they may bring music into their work in a safe and ethical manner. You are the people who support, console, challenge, and encourage children who have suffered a trauma, are emotionally fragile, or have mental health issues that prevent them from fully engaging in life. In our 60-plus years of combined experience as musicians, music therapists, and music therapy educators, we have witnessed many instances in which music makes an immediate difference in how people communicate, socialize, and behave. The judicious use of music can unlock the therapeutic relationship, offer a creative way to work through issues, and provide a path to client success and fulfillment not otherwise possible. Doing this means we have to think about music in a very different way: No longer is it relegated to serving as a background to interactions, or as an aural reflection of love, sadness, yearning, and joy. We can start to think about music as a way to connect with clients in a palpable way. What we want to emphasize here is that you do *not* need to be a trained musician to find therapeutic musical applications to integrate into your work. Following basic clinical and ethical guidelines, it is possible to find effective ways to use music as a therapeutic medium.

Both of us spent our formative years as music therapists working with children who were delayed in communicating, emotionally labile, or otherwise socially or physically impaired. We learned firsthand that music can reach children thought to be minimally capable of response. We have witnessed over and over in our lives, whether with children with autism spectrum disorder, patients in a hospital bed who were seemingly unresponsive, or people with advanced dementia who are no longer able to speak, how music brings people into relationship and into a moment of awareness and interaction. This book is not meant to help the reader learn how to assess or create treatment plans based upon musical engagement, but to identify simple techniques with which to bring music into clinical practice. Knowing how to use music holds the potential to enhance psychotherapy practice in many direct and lasting ways.

The first chapter in the book provides a broad introduction to what music can contribute to therapy. Chapters 2 and 3 together show how to bring music into the therapy room. Chapter 2 describes basic techniques and activities, while Chapter 3 takes this further to show how the clinician can use these strategies in a way that effects positive change. Chapter 4 focuses on children's musical development and describes the powerful role of music in the child's cognitive and emotional development, as well as how to work with children in a developmentally appropriate way. The remaining chapters each provide guidelines for how to intervene musically with a particular population, namely, children with attachment disorders, trauma, and cognitive and behavioral problems, which includes a section on children with autism spectrum disorder.

On a practical note, we decided to use a masculine pronoun when referring to the client and a feminine pronoun when referring to the therapist, for the sake of clarity and simplicity. All client names and identifying information have been changed to ensure anonymity. Also, when writing vignettes we sometimes combined our experiences or made modifications to create stories that are fully anonymized and still remain relevant.

Creating a place for music in your clinical practice is something to be done with planning and also with enthusiasm, for what else can prompt children to play with others in a unified yet individualistic manner that sounds and feels good, or offer a safer way to experience feelings? Our hope is you will read this book and be inspired to incorporate some of its ideas into your practice. Take what works and expand upon it, and please pass some of what you learn on to others.

Acknowledgments

Writing this book has been a rich and rewarding journey. Finding a way to articulate the power of music so it is accessible to a wider audience of clinicians was intense yet exciting. Our collaborative process was surprisingly easy: There were many times when in reading what we had written, we could not tell which of us had written what! Our shared commitment to bringing music to children in need was our touchstone.

We owe a debt of gratitude to Drs. Paul Nordoff, Clive Robbins, and Carol Robbins for blazing a trail of creative music therapy that has transformed the lives of thousands of people. We were in the first training course together at the Nordoff–Robbins Center for Music Therapy at New York University, which was a life-changing experience. There we had the privilege of studying with Drs. Clive and Carol Robbins. Together with a team of like-minded therapists, we learned how to harness the immediacy of music as well as its power to evoke responses and manage emotions; this is the foundation of our careers as clinicians, educators, advocates, and changemakers.

We have had the support and encouragement of many amazing people who have helped us in this book-writing adventure. We are grateful to Rochelle Serwator, our phenomenal editor at The Guilford Press, as well as Dr. Cathy A. Malchiodi, our guide and ally. The entire team at Guilford has been wonderful to work with and has provided professional assistance at every stage of the publication process.

Dr. Barbara Wheeler, thank you for thinking of us and giving us this fantastic opportunity.

To our families—words cannot convey the depth of our appreciation for your love, support, and encouragement. Cyndy, Dean, our children, and grandchildren have been steadfastly loving and understanding. Thank you.

Contents

Chapter 1 Music as a Therapeutic Intervention   1

    Music and Children: A Global Perspective   2
    Music Therapy: Therapeutic Applications of Music   3
    The Experience of Time in Music   6
    Components of Music   10
    Using Music in Clinical Practice   17
    Goals   20
    Benefits   22
    Summary   26
    Recommendations for Practice   27

Chapter 2 Getting Started   29

    Setting Up a Music-Friendly Office   29
    Listening to Instrumental Music and Songs   31
    Singing   32
    Working with Song Lyrics   33
    Using Musical Instruments   37
    Improvisation   39
    Working with the Form and Structure of Music   42
    Working with Imagery and Themes   43
    Music in Group Work   45
    Summary   47
    Recommendations for Practice   47
    APPENDIX 2.1. Suggested Instruments and Equipment   50

Chapter 3 Working with Music as an Agent of Change   57

    Using Music with Different Therapeutic Approaches   58
    Therapeutic Skills   62
    Listening and Being Fully Present   62

How to Talk about Music 65
Music as an Affirmation of the Child 70
Music and Emotion Regulation 71
Using Music to Address Resistance in Therapy 73
Summary 76
Recommendations for Practice 76

Chapter 4 Music in Child Development   79

Typical Development 80
Neuroscience and Music 83
Music and Adolescence 96
Music and Emotions 98
Cultural Lens 99
Summary 102
Recommendations for Practice 102

Chapter 5 Attachment and Attunement in Interpersonal Relationships   106

Theories of Attachment and Attachment-Based Interventions 107
Polyvagal Theory 109
Entrainment 110
Attunement 111
Working with Children with Attachment Problems 115
Working with Parents and Caregivers 121
Working with Groups and Peer Relationships 127
Summary 129
Recommendations for Practice 129

Chapter 6 Trauma and Resilience   132

Processing Trauma through Music 133
Grief and Bereavement 147
Summary 150
Recommendations for Practice 151

Chapter 7 Children with Behavioral, Emotional, and Communication Disorders   157

Music as a Supportive Intervention 158
Interventions for Children with ASD 169
Summary 172
Recommendations for Practice 173

Postscript   177

References   179

Index   195

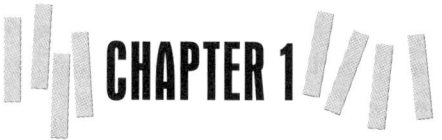

CHAPTER 1

Music as a Therapeutic Intervention

> Music is a world. Every one of us has his own experiences in that world. There are endless depths, infinite varieties and facets of musical experience for the listener, the student, the performer, the composer, and for the therapist.
> —NORDOFF AND ROBBINS (1985, pp. 141–142)

Children are naturally curious and creative. They experience the world as an ever-evolving place of learning, play, and challenge. Music is a natural source of exploration and expression, and an integral component of children's development. In its essence, music is sound shaped into melodies and rhythms that resonate throughout our physical, emotional, and spiritual beings. Whether preverbal, verbal, or nonverbal, music expresses our humanity and serves as a way for us to not only communicate difficult or charged emotions, but also to experience them in a safe and contained way. Mehrabian (2017) found that 90% of human communication is nonverbal in nature, inclusive of tone of voice, body language, eye contact, and emotional tenor. As adults, we tend to focus much of our conscious awareness on spoken language while subconsciously processing the nonverbal cues such as body movements, tone of voice, facial expressions, and degree of eye contact. Young children, especially those with some sort of communication, developmental, social, or cognitive impairment, often live in the nonverbal realm. Reaching them and connecting with them in ways natural to how they perceive the world can be a difficult prospect, yet creative modalities such as music provide an opportunity to be with them in their own worlds. Music gives form and function to the nonverbal state in a way that is relational and immediate. Older children with issues sometimes have trouble accessing and expressing their emotions and thoughts; music can help them give voice to their inner experiences in a manner that is aesthetically appealing, socially valued, and internally rewarding.

Scientific breakthroughs in neuroscience support what people have intuited for millennia: music is a basic part of our human nature, and we are wired to seek out and find meaning in musical experience. Neuroscience researchers are using brain imaging to try to answer the question of what it is about music that makes it so universally valued and loved. They are finding that when we hear pleasurable music, dopamine is released in the brain (Salimpoor, Benovoy, Larcher, Dagher, & Zatorre, 2011). Dopamine is a neurotransmitter that helps control the brain's reward and pleasure centers and is a critical factor in motivating human beings to engage with the world around them. When we even think about having a musical experience that evokes emotion, dopamine enters our system, prompting us to feel more motivated, engaged, and positive (Loxton, Mitchell, Dingle, & Sharman, 2016).

MUSIC AND CHILDREN: A GLOBAL PERSPECTIVE

The development of music in human life parallels humanity's progression toward becoming more and more industrialized. From the whittling of a flute 30,000 years ago to composing music on a computer, each era has its own set of cultural expectations, rules, symbols, and language (verbal and/or written). No matter the form, expression through structured sound has been a constant in our evolution—music and song have been part of human culture since we evolved into sentient and interactive beings. In early human times, the making of tools assured physical survival. Making and playing instruments, along with singing, ensured a creative and social existence. History was once recorded by one generation singing songs about their traditions and experiences to the next generation. Music has also played a vital role in communication—before other means were available, people used drums to send messages to distant villages. Today, we use music as a source of solace and joy, as a way to connect to our inner emotions and to each other: it is both an internal and an external phenomenon. Music's ability to weave together inter- and intra-personal dynamics into one sound is unique and yields rich ground for therapeutic consideration.

All human cultures have language—and music. It is no coincidence that the basic elements of music—rhythm, tempo or pulse, pitch and melody, dynamics, and form—are intimately connected with the production of speech. Spoken language is both rhythmic and melodic. Each sentence has a rhythmic structure, stress patterns, and variations in pitch and inflection which help to communicate its meaning. Singing, a natural activity for children, helps improve auditory perception, processing, and memory. Vocal quality, production of speech sounds, and the learning and retention of language are intrinsic to the experience of singing. Offering predictable rhythmic structures to children with language impairments before being given a prompt increases their ability to successfully process auditory sentences (Bedoin, Brisseau, Molinier, Roch, & Tillmann, 2016). Songs that contain ideas of personal significance to a child are especially effective in stimulating language development. Children's perceptions are sharpened as they learn to distinguish between high and low pitches, fast and slow tempos, and loud and soft dynamics.

Children's songs are part and parcel of every culture's artistic repository. It is widely acknowledged that all cultures use some form of lullabies, or songs designed especially for babies, to help soothe them and get them to sleep. Most lullabies, regardless of the language, use low pitch, slow rise time (the amount of time it takes for a sound to reach its full volume), and a moderate, steady rhythm (Loewy, Stewart, Dassler, Telsey, & Homel, 2013; Smart & Smart, 1978). These characteristics have shown to be soothing for most babies, along with the rhythm of the heartbeat sound.

MUSIC THERAPY: THERAPEUTIC APPLICATIONS OF MUSIC

As humans have developed and evolved, music has become a therapeutic modality in its own right, with its own best practices, research foci, evidence-based approaches, and theoretical orientations. Music therapy is a well-known form of treatment with a rich history and clearly defined standards of practice. Although this volume is written for all professionals working with children, a basic understanding of the field of music therapy is helpful to introduce how music can be used in clinical settings.

Music therapy as a formal discipline in the United States was born after World War I and World War II, when musicians went into hospitals to play for veterans suffering from both physical injuries and psychological trauma (Collins & Fleming, 2017). They found that the veterans responded to music in a way that set it apart from drug treatments, behavioral therapy, and what was known then as convalescence. In 1950, several people formed the National Association for Music Therapy (now the American Music Therapy Association) and began to codify treatment planning and assessment protocols, and the modality began to be integrated into teams as a supportive therapy (Davis & Hadley, 2015). Educational training programs sprang up and from that point on music therapy has grown into an internationally recognized field.

This book is not intended to replace music therapy or sidestep its importance as a therapeutic discipline, for music therapists are specifically trained to recognize and treat many different types of difficulties, and to know how to handle the powerful responses music can evoke in clients. Music can safely express a range of emotions children and adolescents may try to avoid, like sadness, anger, grief, or fear. A song is a finite and time-limited emotional experience, allowing for in-the-moment expression and connection, yet also allowing for a quick distancing from the emotional content when the song ends. When facilitated by a trained therapist, singing becomes a safe, contained, and therapeutic experience. Recognizing when to move in and out of difficult feelings can bring a child a sense of reliability and steadiness not otherwise possible and is an area in which music therapists are highly trained.

The book *Music in Therapy,* edited by E. Thayer Gaston and published in 1968, was one of the first texts to identify how music can be used in a clinical setting with children. Clinicians, doctors, psychiatrists, and psychologists were searching for ways to use music to help children with autism, childhood schizophrenia, behavior disorders, and physical and developmental disabilities, and Gaston's book created a foundation for practice. They began to apply to children principles developed in the work with veterans of World War II, since there was little research on children available at that time. Music therapy educators sought to develop theories and find ways to effectively teach principles and practices to an ever-growing number of students who wanted to become music therapists.

The pioneering work of Paul Nordoff and Clive Robbins illuminates the potential of music in working with children. They began their collaboration in 1959 in Great Britain, exploring the effects of music with children with disabilities in both individual and group therapy (Nordoff & Robbins, 1985). They discovered that children respond to types of music not usually considered suitable for them, such as music with dissonance or unfamiliar scales. For example, a young boy described as regressed and psychotic responded calmly and positively to one type of scale, but cried when he heard music in a scale that contained different tones. Something in the music was clearly affecting him emotionally.

Nordoff and Robbins (1985) were struck with music's power to alter a person's mood and change behavior. They also learned that every child reacts differently to music. Some are drawn to melody, others to rhythm; some intuitively grasp musical form (e.g., phrases, cadences, or endings) while others are less organized. Music is in no way prescriptive; rather, each child responds in his own unique fashion. Using a process of trial and error, they sought to identify music for each child that would elicit a response, using a wide variety of scales and styles. The way a child reacts to music improvised for him creates what they called a "musical portrait." They believed that each individual has his own way of living in the world of music, and that music could help in assessing needs and potentialities: "Communication begins by matching a child's inner condition with music" (Nordoff & Robbins, 1985, p. 40).

Further, Nordoff and Robbins (2007) discovered that the *way* children naturally make music reflects their inner life and struggles; it is a window into their world. Analyzing children's use of tempo (fast vs. slow) and dynamics (loud vs. soft) along a continuum yields valuable information about their emotional states and personality characteristics. Nordoff and Robbins (1985) viewed drum beating as a means of communication, and the way a child beats a drum as an aid in diagnosis. The child's range of playing and flexibility—the ability to easily move between fast and slow tempos, or loud and soft volume—is another indication of mental health. Children facing emotional or developmental challenges tend to be inflexible and to play at the extremes of the continuum—very soft or very loud, very fast or very slow (Nordoff & Robbins, 2007).

A child who has been traumatized may play rigidly, perhaps only in one tempo, or only loud or soft. He may sing using only a very narrow range of tones, or even in a monotone. His playing may be disorganized and he may have trouble regulating himself. He may seem to get "stuck," repeating a rhythmic pattern or phrase without variation, and be unable to develop a musical idea. By helping a child achieve greater flexibility in music, we help him discover new possibilities and ways of thinking about himself. For example, he may come to realize that he is a person who can not only play the drum so loudly and angrily that he drowns out all other sounds, but he can also play softly and allow himself to feel more tender emotions and take in the sounds of others.

Nordoff and Robbins (2007) compared healthy and unhealthy aspects of playing fast, slow, loud, and soft. They found that characteristics of what they called "normal" music experience contrasted with characteristics that are determined by a child's condition or pathology (i.e., developmental disability or emotional disturbance). For example, in normal musical experience, playing in a fast tempo might indicate playfulness, joyfulness, or happy excitement. On the other hand, fast playing might suggest nervousness, overexcitement, or obsessiveness. Playing slowly might communicate thoughtfulness, calmness, or deliberateness. Alternatively, it might convey insecurity, confusion, or lethargy. Loud playing can express animation, eagerness, or confidence, or it may reflect frustration, aggression, or lack of impulse control. And soft playing might express carefulness, delicacy, or suspense in a healthy child, and fear, apathy, or lack of awareness in a troubled child. In whatever way the child plays, the act of creating music brings him into the present moment.

THE EXPERIENCE OF TIME IN MUSIC

Music affects the human brain in a way that no other stimulus or experience does, engaging many different areas simultaneously in an organized way. It exists in time yet is not bound by societal ideas of seconds, minutes, and hours. As such, music makes inherent sense to children, especially those children who struggle with imposed demands to function within specific timeframes. Some children find it hard to respond quickly to yes/no questions or to end an activity within, say, 5 minutes. Music offers a way for children to internally synchronize their thoughts and actions with their feelings, for it "is intrinsically temporal—it integrates sensory, motor and affective systems in the brain" (Temporal Dynamics Learning Center, n.d., para 1).

Children do not experience time the way adults do (DeRobertis, 2008). Although they learn about time and become acclimated to the demands that the clock imposes on their school and home lives, they live in a more fluid experience of time: "Time is lived for the sake of things, people, and events in the here-and-now; schedules are truly of secondary importance" (DeRobertis, 2008, p. 147). They may abide by compulsory adult schedules yet also retain unbounded, in-the-moment responses to what they see, feel, and hear going on around them.

Time is, in this way, a flexible medium in which interactions, sounds, and the flow of events can expand and contract in accordance with the child's experience of reality. Children live in the moment, and for those children who have distorted or different ways of engaging with the world, their sense of flow seems disjointed when compared to how other people perceive time and the continuous movement of events. Flow is a phenomenon studied in positive psychology and has relevance to our understanding of children and time. Simply considered as the state of being completely involved in an activity for its own sake (Csikszentmihalyi, 1990), this state of consciousness gives rise to a genuine sense of satisfaction. Our sense of flow affects not just how we are in the world, but how we respond to and interact with others. During flow, time passes quickly since attention is on the activity at hand and the sense of self as social actor is lost. Children who are impaired or traumatized, however, may experience the flow of time as an oppressive and frustrating phenomenon, for it can be empty of meaning or full of anticipatory fear. For children who experience loneliness or are under constant threat (e.g., living in an abusive household), time is filled with uncertainty and anxiety, and the present moment is felt to be constricting or even threatening. In order to help a child feel safe in the therapy room, it becomes the therapist's responsibility to be cognizant of the child's experience of time and to try to see the world through his eyes.

When working with children who have an alternative awareness of time and flow, music is well suited to creating a space in which the child and therapist experience flow together. Sears (1968) said:

> The unique structure of music—it exists only through time—requires the individual to commit himself to the experience moment by moment. . . . The necessity for moment-to-moment commitment by the individual rests in the music itself. . . . The extent and rapidity of the commitment can be adjusted to the individual by an appropriate selection of the level of skill required, the length and complexity of the music, and the specific responses required. (p. 35)

Music and this concept of flow intersect: both are invigorating, highly and intrinsically enjoyable phenomenon. Combining music, flow, and the therapeutic relationship creates a dynamic environment conducive to forming relationships based on trust, spontaneity, and enjoyment.

Robbins and Forinash (1991) describe four different levels of time experience that encompass the complexity of time in therapy. We find their work useful in understanding both the therapist's and the client's experience. The first level, *physical time*, is how we normally think about time: measurable and predictable. It is time on a schedule and divided into seconds, minutes, and hours. A child has his therapy session on the same day, at the same time, each week—this is an example of physical time. We have seen many children learn the days of the week simply by the consistency of when they attend therapy sessions, for it is something they look forward to and ask about. Parents and teachers are able to reinforce time as measured by a calendar by emphasizing what day it is, and how many more days before they go to music therapy.

Growth time is the time it takes for growth or development to occur. This varies widely from person to person, and from realm to realm. As an example, a child may grasp mathematical concepts quickly but be slower in picking up social cues. Growth time is progressive, variable, and individualized; the growth time of every human being is unique. Children need time and space in which to explore, discover, play, and grow at their own pace.

Emotional time is related to the intensity of our feelings. A few minutes can seem like hours when we are waiting for an important phone call, or, as the saying goes, time flies when you are having fun. We can become so engrossed in our activity that we completely lose track of time; it is as if time is suspended or no longer exists. Robbins and Forinash write:

> For children in therapy it can be very important to live meaningfully—and purposefully—in Emotional Time in music. The stimulation and pleasure of being actively involved in Emotional Time experiences in music heightens perception and concentration, expands feeling awareness, and lessens fixity of emotional tendencies. It brings to the child–therapist relationship a potential—or actual—closeness or mutuality. (1991, p. 52)

Expressing the emotional content of music is an experience of emotional time and is comparable to the concept of flow.

The fourth level is *creative time,* or *now time.* This is the moment of inspiration, intuition, perception, sudden insight, or understanding. Spontaneity and creativity characterize now time. It is in now time that a person feels most fully alive and whole. At this level, children, who naturally live in the immediacy of the moment, can find "new meanings to life, new capabilities and new experiences of creative human contact" (Robbins & Forinash, 1991, p. 53). As therapists, we try to give our clients experiences of these different levels of time, moving from the lower levels to the higher ones. Music, which is temporal, as opposed to the visual arts, lends itself to providing these varying experiences to children.

VIGNETTE

Jack was a lively, energetic 5-year-old boy who had been diagnosed with autism. He was placed in a special school for children with language and communication problems, yet after 3 months in a structured classroom he was only becoming more frustrated and anxious. He was unable to express himself with words and often resorted to tantrums when he could not effectively communicate what he needed or wanted. He was referred to Mindy, a psychologist, for further evaluation and therapy. Mindy's treatment room was large, and for her first meeting with Jack she put away most of the toys and left several carpet squares and a beanbag chair on the floor. She placed three small drums with mallets as well as an autoharp on the floor. After entering, Jack began to quickly circle the room, lightly touching many of the items on shelves as well as the instruments and beanbag chair. He had a tense energy and would not look at Mindy when she tried to verbally engage him. Suddenly he started to run across the room; Mindy picked up the autoharp, held it on her lap and began to strum it rapidly, switching back and forth between C and F chords. Jack looked over at her, slowed down and smiled briefly, then continued to run. Mindy chanted, "Running, running, running!" over and over. On her fifth time of singing it, she slowed down on the last "running!" then added "And stop!" and stopped strumming the autoharp when Jack was right in front of the beanbag chair. Jack could not help but respond: he looked up at Mindy and jumped into the beanbag chair and started laughing. She laughed along with him, and before he had a chance to get out of the chair she started strumming again, slowly at first and then increasing her speed. Jack got up, jumped up and down excitedly as the music got faster, and when Mindy sang "Running, running, running!" he started running. This began a period of engagement. Jack fell into the beanbag chair when the music stopped, and after a few repetitions Mindy exaggerated the slowing down and speeding up portions, which made Jack laugh. His eye contact increased, his affect brightened, and he played this way for 4 minutes. When Mindy felt the interaction had run its course, on the last "Stop!" she kept strumming the autoharp slowly and softly. She sang the song "Row, Row, Row Your Boat" to help Jack calm down. He lay back in the beanbag chair and relaxed while she sang. When Mindy sang, "Life is but a dream," she slowed the phrase down, leaving a longer gap before singing "dream." During this pause Jack looked up at her, as if waiting for her to finish the phrase. She repeated the phrase and again slowed down, this time even more, before singing "dream." Jack got out of the beanbag chair, came over to her and watched her mouth as she sang. After singing the song twice more, Mindy stood up, put the autoharp on a table, and went over to a couch where she sat with Jack, reading to him and playing with a stuffed animal, before bringing him back to the classroom.

In their next session, the running game was brought back, much to Jack's delight. Mindy experimented with singing "And stop!" at different times, and Jack would run to the beanbag chair every time he sensed the stop was coming so he could jump into the chair. It was as if he was learning how to physically stop himself and gain more control over his body. When Mindy started singing "Row, Row, Row Your Boat" Jack immediately stood up and came to stand in front of her, the autoharp on her knees and between them. When she sang "dream," Jack leaned in close to her and said, very softly, "dream." Together they repeated the song over and over, each time singing "dream" together. Jack leaned in even more so that his forehead was touching Mindy's. She was moved by this interaction and, when she later told Jack's mother about it, his mother tearfully said it was the first time she had been given such positive news from anyone at the school.

In reflecting on these two sessions with Jack, Mindy realized that she had been able to tap into Jack's sense of time, which, in the first session, was fast-moving, fleeting. The running song gave him permission to go at his own pace and run freely, yet also be contained by a firm stop. It was when the running time stopped that Jack seemed to be able to notice Mindy more and interact with her by laughing together. This experience was, she realized, an example of flow: she and Jack were engaged in a deeply satisfying music game that had its own sense of time and excitement. Also, the singing of "dream" together felt as if time was suspended and they were alone in this dreamtime, foreheads touching. Entering a flexible, creative experience of time brought them together and created a bond that was therapeutic and fulfilling.

COMPONENTS OF MUSIC

Music comprises the elements of rhythm, melody, and harmony that, when taken separately, have their own sound and character, yet when put together create an aural experience that can evoke emotion and memory. It is similar to how a textile artist will take strands of thread that differ in width, color, and texture, and weave a tapestry. Understanding these components is important to knowing how to therapeutically apply them: "Music and its infinitely variable elements can indeed produce vastly varying responses—from activation to catharsis, and on the polar end of the spectrum, from relaxation response to sedation" (Rossetti, 2014, p. 72). It gives us a way to work with sensory responses, lability, physical reactions, and language-processing abilities in an integrative manner.

Often children with social, communicative, or emotional problems have difficulty controlling and understanding their reactions to sharply contrasting music. How they respond to music mirrors their response to changes in events, sounds, and expectations that take place in their lives. Introducing sounds and music that move from loud to soft, slow to fast, and have different types of evocative melodies gives children a means to gain control over their instinctive response. Helping them become more comfortable with changes in music can have positive reverberations in other areas of their lives. When considering what forms or styles of music are most suited for a situation, there are factors such as age, gender, and culture to account for. In one study, music from various cultures elicited similar emotional responses, while gender differences more typically influenced listening preferences and affective responses (Upadhyay, Shukla, Tripathi, & Agrawal, 2017). Upadhyay et al. (2017) studied how personality, emotion, gender, and psychosocial context interacted in the listening preferences of adolescents and found that girls tend to prefer more romantic and slow-paced songs, while boys have a preference for fast-moving and louder songs. This information is not meant to be prescriptive, but rather serve as a guide for psychotherapists working with children and teens, for music choices are also culture-bound—even young children prefer the company of people who know the same songs they do (Soley & Spelke, 2016). Whether differences in musical inclinations are due to inborn genetic factors or are culturally determined is an active area of research and discussion. With this in mind, an understanding of the specific components of music is helpful when considering introducing music in a therapeutic environment.

Melody

A melody carries the emotional expression of a piece of music; the rise, fall, and leaps in a melody capture nuances of emotion. One melodic line can take us through feeling happy, to wistful, to content. Studies show that melodies we learn early in our lives, like the "The ABC Song" or those associated with religious rituals, stay with us throughout our lifetime, through illness and age. They become imbedded in the limbic area of our brains as implicit memory and are retrievable even in the deep fog of advanced dementia (Beer, 2017). People who have advanced dementia can still sing a song they learned decades ago, and in remembering the melody reconnect to some part of their younger self. For children who are unable to use words to express their inner world and needs, a melody gives them a form to hold on to that captures the essence of their feeling.

The melody of a piece of music is often its main identifier, especially in popular music. Songs played on the Top 40 radio stations, for example, have catchy themes that are immediately recognizable and prompt listeners to sing along. Being aware of the effects a melody has is important if you are to bring music into a session: Does it have a falling effect, thus evoking a sad or contemplative mood? Or does it push upward, bringing a sense of hope or joy? A therapist can create short melodies that support or reflect a child's mood or actions, relying on these general effects of melody. For example, if the child you are working with is in a bright, happy mood, you could sing "Marcus is smiling" with a melody that moves up the scale. This reinforces Marcus' demeanor in a playful and inviting manner. You are able to affirm the child's mood in a way that does not overwhelm him or cause him to feel like he is being observed and somehow judged.

The distance between two notes in a melody is known as an interval. While listening to music is a deeply personal experience, characteristics of certain intervals are widely accepted. An octave is the distance from C to the next C, for example, and has a feeling of space. The direction of the interval is also significant. Think of the first two notes of the song "Somewhere over the Rainbow" (Arlen & Harburg, 1939): *some-where*—the rising octave has a strong, uplifting feeling. If the interval moved in the other direction—from high to low—it would have a very different feeling. A tritone (also called an augmented fourth or diminished fifth) consists of two tones that are three whole steps apart. This interval (e.g., E to B flat) sounds tense, unfinished, and unsettled. Sometimes ambulance sirens blast this interval, as its dissonance grabs people's attention and warns them to get out of the way. In medieval times, the church banned the tritone from its music, calling it the devil's music. If the tritone is enlarged by just a half step, it becomes a perfect fifth, an interval characterized by stability and a feeling of groundedness.

Rhythm

The original rhythm for all human beings is the heartbeat. It is estimated that we hear our mother's heartbeat 20 million times before we are born. Some believe infants in the womb do not necessarily hear these muffled beats, but rather feel them through the amniotic fluid (Page, 1995; Quinn & Knoerlein, 2016). Either way, rhythm is a sensed phenomenon, ingrained in our physiological systems, in our own heartbeat and breath patterns. Our internal rhythms of heartbeat, respiration, and blood pressure all indicate levels of health. Rhythm is also a term used in social contexts, carrying with it a sense of whether someone is in synchrony with events, emotions, or experiences happening in or around them. For example, saying "I am out of sync today" implies that there is a mismatch between inner experience and outer behavior; there is something "off" that prevents a person from feeling fully present or functional.

Focusing on rhythm when in session with a child "can be an effective way to develop both stability and the ability to encounter, absorb, and create change" (John Haek, personal communication, January 8, 2018). When a person is fully engaged rhythmically, he is "in the groove," acting and responding in the moment to stimuli and interactions. When a steady pulse is provided to serve as the foundation for rhythmic play, a sense of predictability, stability, and familiarity is created that can then support the development of patterns. The patterns can be simple or complex; having the foundation allows the patterns to be safely developed and become more intricate and interactive.

John Haek, a music theory professor, says, "Sound itself comes alive with rhythm, sound *is* rhythm: the vibrations that create sound are rhythmic. The rhythmic components of melody are immediately and powerfully communicative" (personal communication, June 6, 2017). When responding to music that has a strong rhythmic drive through sound or movement, children become more spontaneous; they intuitively sense what is coming next and in anticipating it, open themselves to coordinating their thoughts, emotions, and physical responses so they can be even more fully engaged.

Timbre

When someone plays a D note on an oboe, it sounds very different from the sound a viola makes when playing the same note. The difference in the quality of the sound is referred to as timbre. How a single note sounds to us depends upon many different characteristics such as whether the instrument is made from wood or metal, yet ultimately, how we hear music is a psychological phenomenon. The human brain processes sound and categorizes it according to its complexity of tone, and each instrument, including the human voice, emits a different combination of frequencies. This leads us into a discussion of what instruments to choose when working with children. The differing timbres of instruments yield very different effects: you might offer a tambourine to a child who rejects it immediately yet is eager to pick up and play a medium-sized hand drum. In your opinion there may not be much difference between a tambourine, with its drum skin and metal jingles, and the drum, yet the child clearly does not like the higher-pitched and sharp sound of the tambourine, preferring the lower tone of the drum.

Another aspect of timbre is that it "plays an important role in the cognition of musical patterns" (Hodges & Sebald, 2011, p. 146). This comes into play especially in group work, for if you choose instruments that have similar timbres, such as various floor drums (e.g., tubano and djembe), the overall sound will blend and distinct instruments or rhythmic patterns may not be able to be heard or identified. If your goal is for each child to have a unique experience in group music making and to blend individual voices into a group sound, you will want to choose instruments that have contrasting timbre such as triangle, floor drum, soprano xylophone, maracas, and egg shakers. Awareness of timbre will guide you in choosing what instruments to place in a therapy room, knowing the potential effects of individual and blended sounds.

Harmony

When two or more tones or melodies combine, harmony is created. Harmony gives profundity and richness to music. Chords are created, and the harmony that comes from chordal progressions gives a piece of music its emotional depth, or, as is the case with children's music, its sense of playfulness and lightness. Some chords are consonant, meaning that the sounds mix together to create a pleasing sensation. Other chords are dissonant, meaning that the sounds are discordant, or seem to clash. Whether we hear a harmony as consonant or dissonant is subjective, based on the sounds we are accustomed to hearing. An unfamiliar chord may seem dissonant to us at first, but once we become used to it, it sounds more consonant. Consonant harmonies often instill peaceful, relaxing feelings. A therapist can use consonant harmonies to support a child who is feeling mellow, or, alternatively, when trying to transform the mood of a child who may be upset or agitated. Dissonant harmonies can be stimulating or jarring, so a therapist might want to use dissonant harmonies when she wants to "shake things up" and provide a new challenge.

Melody and harmony work in combination to generate movement and direction in music; tensions are created and resolved through the movement of notes and chords. When listening to a piece of music with a client, being able to identify how harmony affects the listener is a skill that can be developed. If you, as a clinician, verbalize that a piece of music has lush harmonies, this is a point of potential discussion with your client: Do you both hear this? How does the rich sound affect each of you? When talking about favorite movie themes with preadolescent boys and girls, we have been struck by their choice of songs from *Star Wars* and *Superman*: both theme songs are dense with harmonies that on the surface seem perhaps too complicated for this age group yet hold great appeal for them.

Dynamics

How loud or soft music is determines its dynamic level. When working with young children or those unable to engage in a verbal discussion, being aware of dynamics is an important part of choosing an appropriate song or piece of music to play. For example, if a client is in an agitated state, choosing a soothing lullaby to listen to might have an opposite effect and aggravate him. The softness of the song may be too far removed from the child's internal state and cause even more agitation.

From a psychological perspective, the volume of music is more than just its loudness or softness; it is a range of aural experiences between two widely divergent ends of the auditory spectrum. Working with dynamics and helping a child become more comfortable with sounds on either end of this spectrum can at the same time develop flexibility and increase tolerance of loud sounds (Ilie & Thompson, 2006). Exploring contrasts helps children increase their sense of control, for moving from making loud to soft (or soft to loud) sounds naturally expands their range of expression and internal regulation. Often, children will cover their ears when there are loud, or even moderate or soft, sounds in the environment. Parents sometimes report to us that their child has a sensitivity to sound. Yet when given the opportunity to beat a drum or crash a cymbal, these same children will play loudly, with great abandon. It appears that it is not the volume itself that causes distress, but rather the unpredictability of the sound. When the child himself is in control of making the sounds, he can tolerate a wider range of dynamics. In this situation the goal becomes helping the child become more comfortable with sounds created by others.

Being able to move between playing loud and soft and have some control over how loudly to play also reflects inner emotional states. Chau and Horner (2015) found that introducing deliberate changes in dynamics gave children a way to talk about their emotions. For example, loud music is often associated with being angry and soft sounds with being shy. It can be easier to talk about anger or shyness in the context of a piece of music, and from there to explore individual responses and thoughts. Interestingly, being happy is minimally affected by changes in dynamics (Chau & Horner, 2015).

Form

Musical form refers to the overall structure or plan of a piece of music, including phrases (musical sentences or ideas) and the organization of different sections. Many children in treatment experience an internal sense of chaos, disorganization, and lack of structured or predictable response to events and interactions. Building the child's capability to integrate and respond to internal feelings as well as the environment is crucial to the success of therapy, yet it can be difficult to determine how to best achieve these goals through music. Understanding form in music can help therapists approach their work in a more intentional and goal-directed manner. Each piece of music has a distinct form: it may have one dynamic with minimal changes in phrasing, such as in songs like "Baa, Baa, Black Sheep," or it may have contrasting sections built into it, like the ones built into the verses of "The Wheels on the Bus" that have different motions, tempos, and dynamics. If you are seeking to build a sense of stability and continuity with a young client, you may choose the former song, while if you are working toward the child tolerating and adapting to shifts in dynamics and speed, you might choose the latter song.

There are several key elements when considering form in music with children, such as repetition, starts and stops, predictability, and layers of complexity. Children learn through repetition, yet repetition can become tedious when presented as a learning activity. Introduce a song that has repetition, however, and a child might sing and be engaged for much longer periods of time. Adults may get bored by the seemingly endless verses of "The Bear Went Over the Mountain," yet children delight in the variety of scenes that can be enacted. Predictability in music ensures consistency, helps a child feel secure in his knowledge of a song, and can increase a relaxation response. Yet an element of surprise, such as the "pop!" in "Pop! Goes the Weasel," injects a sense of heightened awareness and interest and can serve to keep a child engaged (Rossetti, 2014). Working within the given structure of a song offers a feeling of stability and a way for a young client to safely participate in a form of creative play.

USING MUSIC IN CLINICAL PRACTICE

Offering creative encounters through music provides an alternative to the typical emphasis of many treatment approaches on verbalizing emotions. When engaging in inventive forms of play, children forge new realities, new ways of thinking and feeling about issues. Making up songs, tapping new rhythms that reflect their internal rhythms, and rhyming are spontaneous acts that express internal reality in a playful way. Children who have not yet learned how to use words to express their emotions can hold on to a melody, a line of a song, or a rhythmic motif that captures their feeling. When music matches the child's emotional state, he feels acknowledged and understood.

When added to the client–therapist relationship and used in a therapeutic way, music becomes a third presence in the room, something to talk about, refer to, and also use as a way to tap into wells of emotion not accessible through words alone. Music can be both a personal and a shared experience. Giving clients a way to experience music that is suited to their developmental ability, culture, and maturity allows them to feel things they might not otherwise feel, and gives you, the clinician, a way to talk about these feelings in a way that does not feel potentially intrusive. Asking a child "What did you feel while listening to that piece of music?" is very different from asking "What are you feeling right now?" It is less threatening for many children who may not have the words or ability to directly voice their innermost feelings. We discuss how to approach listening to and processing music more in Chapter 4.

Building Confidence in Using Music

In speaking with therapists who work with children in varying settings, we have heard again and again the sentiments "I'm not a musician": "I don't know how to use music"; and "I'm no good at music." Hesitancy to use music in a therapeutic way can stem from never having played an instrument or having only played one as a child, or a lack of confidence in one's musical abilities. In the past, music was considered as natural to being human as breathing and people were more spontaneous in singing or playing. In some countries this is still a fundamental belief, yet in Western culture music has become something deified, a pursuit only for the gifted. This tenet holds many practitioners back from tapping into a direct line to children's inner states and strengths. The inner critic's voice creates a block to working in a fuller, more spontaneous way. Yet music, when used in a direct and simplified manner, can be a potent clinical tool.

Before embarking on the journey of using music in your practice, it is essential to take a close look at your own assumptions and reactions. When you imagine using music, do you relax and think "Yes, I'd like to do this!" or do you worry and think "I'd like to but I've been told I have no musical ability"? It is actually very rare that someone has *no* musical ability. We believe that we all respond to music and have the capacity to harness its power for directed goals. Right now, you can use music effectively, in some way, in your practice. In this book you will find the tools to learn how: we start from a place of confidence and assurance that you have the underlying skills and sensitivities necessary to figuring out exactly how you will implement the suggestions you find here. Picking up a hand drum, for example, and becoming comfortable in playing it, varying rhythms, tempos, and dynamics, is well within your reach. Listen to music from different cultures and play along. It may feel artificial or awkward at first, yet this is a way to build your skill level. Practicing will most assuredly lead to greater abilities. It is all too common in American culture that we are given the message that few people are musicians. The truth is we are all musical—in reading this book you are taking a step toward opening up the world of music to not only your clients, but also yourself. Your hesitancy to use music may very well be something you learned from others, and you can now let it begin to fade away. We think it is no coincidence that the word "play" has one meaning of engaging in child-like explorations, and another of making music. Playing is a way of experiencing the world that asks us to let the critical voice stay silent.

Identifying Personal Preferences

Assessing your own preferences and musical tastes is an important part of being able to separate your natural inclinations from what a therapeutic situation requires. We encourage you to take some time and complete the following exercise. Following these steps and writing out your responses will give you a deeper understanding of your own musical preferences. It can also help you become more aware of the potential for transference and countertransference that is present in musical experiences.

1. What music do you tend to listen to? Are there certain songs or types of music you listen to when you are feeling happy, sad, lonely, or frustrated?
2. Think of a time when you were feeling sad or grieving over a loss. Did you turn the radio off when some songs came on and turn the volume up for others? Which songs were they?
3. Write down five songs or pieces of music that you like to listen to when feeling low.
4. Put these into a playlist and listen to all five without stopping. What are you feeling after listening to these pieces? Are you surprised by your response?
5. Repeat Steps 3 and 4, this time focusing on songs or pieces of music that you like to listen to when feeling happy or content.
6. Compare the two sets of notes and identify any similarities in what the music brought up for you. Did listening to these sets of music help you experience the emotions of sadness or happiness in a different way? What were the differences?

Another exercise is to identify the music you listen to while driving in the car or commuting to work. For 2 weeks, mentally note what you listen to as you are traveling. When you arrive at your destination, take a few moments to write down what you listened to and why you think you were drawn to that music on that particular day. How closely connected are your musical choices to what is going on in your life? Are there patterns that emerge? Do your choices vary day to day, or do they tend to stay the same? Are there certain genres (like classic rock, new age, classical, or world music) that you prefer?

The purpose of doing these exercises is to be able to articulate the music you like and why. When you are working with a client, being transparent and honest about music is essential. Sharing your own tastes in music can serve as an indirect form of self-disclosure that must be evaluated, but, by and large, talking about the music you like with a young client is another way to establish a deeper sense of trust.

GOALS

Primary goals in child psychotherapy revolve around helping children develop healthy attachments, learn to regulate their emotions, cope with the effects of trauma, and become more integrated into their social world (Lieberman & Van Horn, 2011). This can be invigorating and also challenging work. A psychotherapist must rely upon her own skills and experiences to forge connections, create opportunities for change, and interpret results. Integrating music into a clinical psychotherapy practice with children allows a psychotherapist to access an alternative route to common goals. Music brings a transdisciplinary perspective, for it concomitantly works within the domains of emotional, social, communicative, physical, behavioral, and developmental functioning. For example, engaging in playing drums with a child to strengthen a therapeutic bond involves activating pro-social behaviors like maintaining eye contact and interacting with others. It also develops physical coordination, addresses emotional goals by increasing feelings of self-control and self-esteem, encourages healthy behaviors (e.g., modulating responses and controlling impulses) to create satisfying music, and engages both sides of the child's brain, thereby supporting and enhancing neuroplasticity and brain development.

It is helpful to have a list of general goals to consider when incorporating music into therapy sessions with children. These are intended to frame some of the more in-depth work to come in later chapters. The goals presented here are a preliminary list that we encourage you to expand and add to.

1. *Self-regulation.* Music is a naturally engaging and activating force that children respond to with movements, words, and vocalizations. When children express themselves in music it feels good: they are supported and encouraged by the music. The internal sensations of pleasure and connection motivate them to control impulses that might otherwise derail the musical process, and also to work to fit their responses into the music's structure. For example, a 9-year-old child who is unable to control her angry outbursts when asked to interact with other children might be motivated to control her anger after being told she has a lovely singing voice and invited to join the school choir. A therapist could work with the child's desire to participate successfully in the choir and help her gain better control of her emotions; the child's positive motivation can help her overcome her tendency to get angry in order to accept the musical direction necessary to being a choir member.

2. *Increase social engagement.* By participating in a dyadic or group music intervention, a child is practicing social skills. Every child's musical role is important to the integrity of the piece and so each will want to conform to the demands of waiting, taking turns, and fully engaging when it is appropriate to do so. The previous example of the child engaging in choral singing holds significance here. From another social perspective, children also make friends in music. Developing friendships is crucial to becoming a healthy adult, and musical exchanges foster friendly interactions based on cooperation and respect. For children who did not have healthy attachments with adults early on, engaging in musical play can re-create these.

3. *Cognitive abilities.* Learning words to a new song, waiting to play or sing until the music requires it, and deciding how much volume or intensity to put into the music are comparable to developing cognitive skills of memory, sequencing, and decision making. These skills are intrinsic components of playing a piece of music that is satisfying to listen to. Research indicates that children who learn how to play music at an early age have greater amounts of gray matter in their brains, and that the resultant enhanced brain development has life-long beneficial effects (Rogenmoser, Kernbach, Schlaug, & Gaser, 2018).

VIGNETTE

Mary was an 18-month-old child living in a pediatric intensive care unit. She had been moved there from the neonatal intensive care unit when she was 5 months old, as she had a severe congenital heart condition that required constant monitoring. Mary's development was slow, and the nurses did what they could to foster her growth. They took her outside on sunny days, talked and played with her, and brought in age-appropriate toys. The reality of her life, however, was that she was growing up in an environment that required suppression of all types of noises and was sterile in terms of visual stimuli. She was growing physically, yet her social skills were limited by the environment and her ability to create vocal sounds was impaired by the fact that she was on a respirator.

A child life specialist, Brent, quickly noticed her lack of social development. He had received some training in using music with young children and decided to try some of the techniques with Mary. During the first session, a nurse held Mary up in a sitting position on a floor mat while Brent held her hands and clapped with her to the beat of "Row,

Row, Row Your Boat." This seemed to energize Mary, and she smiled at him as he felt her put some of her own effort into the clapping.

When Brent next visited Mary, she was sitting up on the floor mat again, this time held up by a physical therapist (PT). Mary had her head down and appeared to be passively allowing her body to be manipulated. The PT, Yulia, invited Brent to co-treat and so he again sat on the mat and faced Mary. Yulia was working on turning from side to side by twisting Mary's trunk, creating a back and forth motion. Brent sang "The Wheels on the Bus" and Yulia quickly matched the pace and rhythm of her movements with Mary's to the rhythm of the song. Mary picked her head up and looked at Brent and smiled a wide, happy smile. Yulia said she could feel more strength in Mary's core muscles and she seemed to be engaging with the movement, and asked Brent to keep singing. On a hunch, Brent began to sing the gospel song "This Little Light of Mine" in an upbeat tempo and Yulia modified the turning motions to fit the new song. The second time Brent sang it through (repetition is important for children), Yulia paused the movements, allowing Mary to sit still. Mary did not move at first, then suddenly picked her shoulders up, shrugged them, and turned her body slightly from side to side: "She's dancing!" one of the nurses exclaimed. Indeed, Mary was moving and turning slightly all by herself, and then began to vocalize an "Ah" sound over and over. This was the first time in her short life that Mary initiated a movement and vocalization without being prompted by an adult or by an internal sensation of pain or discomfort. She organized her body movements in response to the song and engaged with Brent vocally—this was a breakthrough of self-determination and involvement.

Brent continued working with Mary to strengthen and further develop her skills, and Mary was more active and involved not only in the sessions, but in all aspects of her life. She became more animated with the staff members on the unit and was observed to laugh more. Within 8 weeks she was fitted with glasses that helped her to see better and a foster family had stepped forward to take her home. Brent was told repeatedly by staff members that his work seemed to have sparked in Mary a desire to interact and engage with the world.

BENEFITS

Music has rewards that are both immediate and long-lasting. For a child who has difficulty forming positive attachments to adults or other children, becoming engaged in musical play can serve as the confidence booster necessary for taking the first steps toward trusting another person. When playing a drum along to a favorite song, singing karaoke-style, or improvising what it feels like to be outside on a rainy day, for example, the children's imaginations are activated; their emotions must be controlled so they serve to enhance, not detract from, the music; and they must be sensitive to the music the therapist is playing. We will discuss these benefits in more detail in Chapter 2.

Music naturally evokes emotions and children instinctively respond to the feelings associated with the upward curve of a melody, the driving rhythm of a drum beat, or the harmonies in a sad song. Choosing songs and instruments to play that either match or hold the potential to shape emotional expression creates opportunities in which children can actively participate and express their emotions in a safe and contained manner. When emotions are touched upon in this way, children often have responses that indicate increasing empathy; engaging in group music play tends to strengthen empathy even more (Rabinowitch, Cross, & Burnard, 2013).

Music does not automatically evoke specific images, feelings, or memories, but rather prompts children to respond with their imagination. The stories, characters, events, and ideas that come out of musical engagement offer glimpses into the inner world of the child. Their imaginal play reflects how they integrate experiences and interactions.

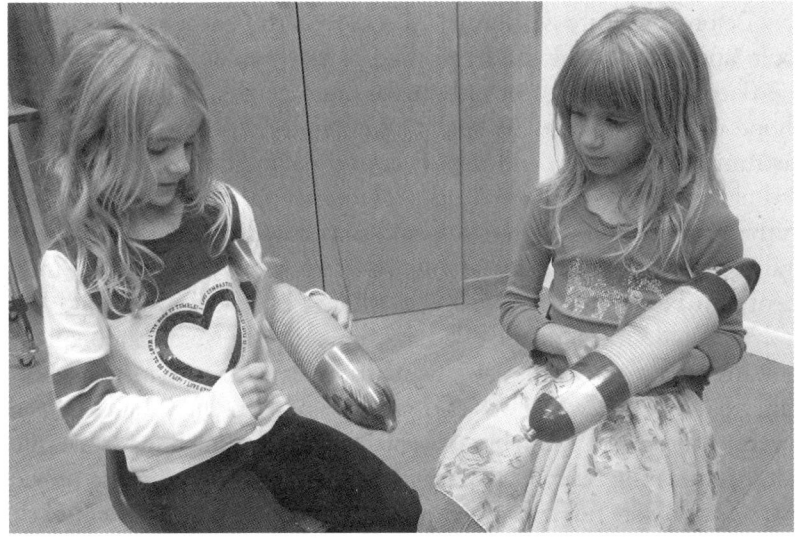

Two girls playing guiros

VIGNETTE

Raul, 7 years old, was referred to a child psychotherapist, Vera, for noncompliance issues arising at home and at school. His parents, teachers, and school officials had reached a point of frustration, for none of the goals, boundaries, or expectations they had for him had any effect on his unwillingness to sit still in class and not constantly disrupt by talking, throwing paper at children around him, looking out the window while he was supposed to be taking tests, and mocking other students. He had been evaluated for emotional, social, and physical issues, yet nothing conclusive had been established. The psychologist at the school suggested he might be developing attention-deficit/hyperactivity disorder (ADHD).

Vera was skilled in verbal and play therapy techniques and began her sessions with Raul by offering him a choice of ways to play: sand tray, puppets, cars, and clay. For the first two sessions he chose to play with the cars and would intensely focus on racing them around the room. Vera attempted to join him in this play by mirroring some of his play and parallel playing with a different car. For the most part, Raul calmly ignored her play and avoided answering her questions about why he chose a certain car, or where he might go in the car if he could go anywhere. She felt he was, in effect, building a wall that shut her out. In her intake interview with Raul's parents they had not indicated that music was a particular favorite activity for him, but his lack of engagement and growing resistance to her presence warranted, she felt, a new approach.

Before the third session, Vera removed the cars from the therapy room and covered the sand tray. She placed two large hand drums on the floor, along with a set of bongos, four egg shakers, and a metallophone with two mallets. When Raul entered the room, he noticed the instruments right away and went over to the hand drums, picking one up and playing it. He beat the drum vigorously and rapidly, and then went to the metallophone. Before he could start playing it, Vera stepped over and picked up the mallets, saying, "Let me show you how this instrument can be played. Do you know what it is called?" Raul said "No," and repeated "metallophone" after Vera said the word. She explained how important it was to play this instrument with care in order not to damage it. She knew she was taking a leap of faith here: Raul's behavior at school indicated he might start playing the instrument with the intention of drowning her out, yet her interactions with him in the previous two sessions were not fraught with tension and she hoped she could trust him to cooperate. She played a few notes lightly on the metallophone and asked him if he understood the rules. He replied "Yes." She gave him the mallets and watched as he grasped them and began to play slowly and delicately. He first went up and down the range of notes, and then started to jump around, playing different bars. He settled into a steady tempo and Vera picked up the bongos and began to play the first and third beat, musically supporting his exploration with a steady yet unobtrusive pattern. Inwardly she was surprised when he did not insist she stop playing. Instead he became a little stronger in his play and began to use both mallets, creating intervals. The result was a lush sound that had a dreamlike feel to it, as if it were music being played for a fairy tale. After several minutes the music came to a natural ending point: his became softer and softer, fading away, and Vera mirrored this. She made sure to stop before he did so he had the last note ringing in the air. He looked up at her and whispered, "That was really cool!" Vera agreed, and asked him what it sounded like. Raul responded, "It sounded like magic." Vera said, "Yes, it sounded like a magic story." Raul replied, "Like a wizard in a castle!" From there they stopped playing music and began to construct a story about the wizard, with Raul telling most of it and Vera offering prompts when he became stuck. It turned out that the wizard was very lonely in his castle. He had no friends, no one to eat with. He had these amazing powers, but no one seemed to like him.

Over the next few sessions the story evolved. Raul drew pictures of the castle and the wizard, and with Vera's support played music that matched different parts of the story. In between working on the story Raul would answer some of Vera's questions about school, and he shared that the other children would not sit with him in the lunchroom and called him "freak" on the playground. His actions at school were attempts to reject others before they rejected him, which led to a cycle of negative behavior that was becoming entrenched. In the sixth session, the wizard became angry and cast spells on townspeople that made them afraid and angry. Vera said, "Let's put music to this" and Raul agreed. Together they decided to first play the frustrated and angry wizard, then the townspeople. When it came time to play music about the townspeople, Vera asked him what he imagined they were feeling. He said they seemed afraid and decided to play the metallophone rather than the hand drum, which was his first inclination. He picked out a short melody that had a sad feeling to it, and Vera hummed along, making downward slides with her voice that indicated melancholy. When he finished playing, he paused, then stated, "That's how I feel, too. Sad. Then I get angry." Vera heard this as a potent statement of his true feeling. She asked him, "I wonder if maybe we could just be sad, and not get angry?" She started to hum again, and he began to play the metallophone slowly, thoughtfully. When this piece ended she thanked him for his music. She decided to take a risk, and asked him, "Do you think you could work on not getting angry at school?" Raul sat in silence for a while, and then said, "Yeah, I could try."

In the sessions that followed, the story and accompanying music began to include some friendly visitors; a brother of the wizard whom he really liked came to stay, and they had some wonderful adventures. While this was happening in his psychotherapy sessions, Raul became noticeably calmer at school, disrupting his classroom fewer and fewer times. As he became calmer, his teacher reported, other children started to say "Hi" to him and volunteer to be his work partner on assignments. Things were beginning to shift.

After 12 sessions, Vera felt Raul was more able to control his actions. She suggested to him that they have two more sessions and he agreed. She then asked him if he would like to draw parts of the story and record some of the music that went along with it. Raul was eager to do this. During his final session, he invited his parents to come into the room. He and Vera told the story, complete with pictures and music, in which the wizard transformed from a lonely and angry person to someone who was able to help the townspeople and animals around him. Catastrophes were averted and a couple of "really bad people" magically became happy and nice.

Raul's parents were thrilled that he was able to come to terms with school and felt pride in what he was able to create. When Vera met with them to review the goals, it was clear he was learning how to stay calm and reduce his angry outbursts. He seemed less sad and began to connect socially with other children. Vera felt that music offered a nonverbal way for Raul to release emotions and help regulate his behaviors. He also developed a greater capacity to empathize with the characters he created, reflecting his growing ability to understand what others around him were feeling.

SUMMARY

Music speaks to the whole child and offers therapists a way of accessing strengths and motivations not otherwise engaged: "There is a lived and living affinity between what we call the 'laws of music'—in all their cultural diversity—and the totality of our spiritual, emotional, mental, and physical evolving" (Robbins, 2005, p. 55). In this chapter we answered the question "Why music?" and offered ways clinicians can begin to understand how to use this powerful creative form, beginning with personal assumptions and fears, and expanding into practice.

RECOMMENDATIONS FOR PRACTICE

The work with both Mary and Raul demonstrates how a clinician can incorporate music into her therapeutic work. With Mary, Brent introduced simple children's songs to evoke physical and social responses, while Vera used instruments to enhance and amplify the drama Raul created with his characters. There are many ways clinicians working with children can begin to use music in their sessions. The suggestions below are general guidelines.

- Sing and/or vocalize when working with young children. Very often children are better able to hear and understand verbal exchanges when they are sung. If you think you are not able to sing in tune, vocalize sounds using vowels: ah, ay, ee, eye, oh, and ooh are all sounds anyone can make and that children are drawn to imitating. Singing changes how children hear words: when Brent sang "Row, Row, Row Your Boat" to Mary, she instinctively responded when the words alone did not motivate her.
- Co-treat when possible. Working alongside physical therapists, occupational therapists, and speech–language pathologists and bringing music into a session reinforces their strategies in a way that feels natural to children. For example, when an occupational therapist is working on finger dexterity, helping the child act out "Where Is Thumbkin?" reinforces the use of individual fingers. We offer a caveat here: observe the child carefully and be aware of when to stop the music. Stop at the first sign of distress or anxiety, for without training in music therapy it can be difficult to assess when music might overstimulate a child.
- Follow your intuition. Both Vera and Brent had a moment where intuition sparked an idea for a therapeutic intervention, and they both followed it. Vera brought in the metallophone and sensed it would be okay to let Raul know how to play the instrument, that he would not damage it. Brent had a sense that singing a more upbeat and lively

song might connect with Mary, and indeed it did spur her to begin dancing.

- Storytelling. With older children like Raul, creating a personal story or adapting a familiar story is a way to form powerful metaphors for their lives. Adding music to the story adds to the challenge as well as the internalized feeling of control and success. The tale takes on an even greater dramatic feeling and becomes something to share with others (see Chapter 5).

- Honor your accomplishments. It can be easy to discount a therapeutic success as possibly being a one-off event or specific to only one child, yet taking some extra time to document fully what you did, why you did it, and the results you observed gives you a foundation to build upon. For example, Brent took time at home to write out his experiences with Mary as a narrative, inclusive of his own responses and reactions. When he finished he read it to his partner, who exclaimed, "That is a beautiful story." Brent was struck by this comment and so continued to add to the story. When Mary went home, Brent shared the story with the nurses who had cared for her. They were touched by how he had included many of their statements as well as observations of how loving they were in their care of Mary.

- For therapists who do not have a high level of confidence in actively making music, choosing songs that reflect emotional qualities and have a range of tempos, dynamics, and melodic changes can be a way to work with a child's ability to identify and regulate feelings. You can also consider making up short songs about being happy, sad, or angry that include personal facts about the child's life.

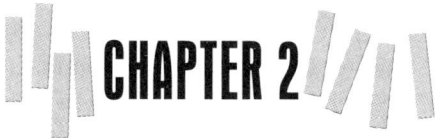

Getting Started

*Music captures children's immediate attention,
so when the music starts, so do the children!*
—HOLCK AND JACOBSEN (2017, p. 159)

Finding ways to bring music into clinical practice can enliven and enrich the therapeutic process. It can also be intimidating, especially if you do not consider yourself to be a musician. In this chapter, we describe what you will need to do to set up an office equipped for working with music and provide an overview of basic techniques that will be discussed further later in the book. We include definitions and examples of common techniques, many of which are used in music therapy and can be modified for use by other clinicians. The chapter provides clear parameters for knowing how and when to bring music into treatment and how to work with children in a manner that is both safe and respectful of their musical process. Chapter 3 goes into more detail about how to use music to facilitate therapeutic change.

SETTING UP A MUSIC-FRIENDLY OFFICE

There are several issues to consider when setting up an office that is conducive to active music making. One is the size of the room—a child with poor boundaries and self-regulation may find it overwhelming to be in a very large space. He may feel insecure or confused about where to go and how to move his body through the area. A smaller room may provide a comforting feeling of containment that leads to the child feeling safe in the environment. On the other hand, children listening to music may want to move to the music or even move around the room. Ideally the space should be large enough to allow children to move around freely while feeling safe and contained. The room should also be of a size to comfortably hold equipment and instruments.

Within the office, avoid having a large number of objects in the room. Open shelves lined with books, toys, or instruments may be distracting. A child may not be able to choose an activity or instrument if too many are available, or he may flit from one to another without being able to engage with any in a meaningful way. A closet or closed cabinet can be helpful to keep instruments out of reach or sight of the child while remaining easily accessible to you. Likewise, it is often best to offer just two or three instrument choices rather than present a basket filled with them.

The office should provide a comfortable place for listening to music with the child or adolescent. Provide several options for children to choose from, like whether to sit on a couch or on large pillows or a beanbag chair on the floor. Some children are better able to focus when they are lying down and feel grounded by the sensation of their bodies being supported by the floor.

A child's safety is the highest priority. Instruments must be stable and soundly constructed to avoid falling over, breaking, or causing injury. If a child tends to mouth objects, avoid instruments that might cause harm, such as ones that have small bells that can be bitten off. Though exploration in sound making should be encouraged, instruments must be used safely. For example, a child should be seated or lying down when playing a blowing instrument. It is dangerous for a child to be running around the room while blowing a reed horn since there is a risk of falling and injuring his mouth.

The sound environment must also be taken into consideration. How much ambient noise is there in the room? It can be difficult to achieve a peaceful silence when there are loud street noises outside or air conditioners humming inside. Certain kinds of lighting create an audible hum that can be distracting, so you may want to dim or turn off some of the lights. Do sounds reverberate throughout the room, making those of even modest volume seem uncomfortably loud? Perhaps curtains might help absorb some of the sound, or even some soundproofing tiles on the ceiling or walls. The therapist must also be aware of the safety of the volume of the music. Listening to loud music can permanently damage the sensitive inner structures of the ear; rock musicians are notoriously hard of hearing at an earlier age than is typical due to the constant loudness of the music they perform (Morata, 2007). It is also important to find an office where you will not disturb people around you. Concern that the music will disrupt someone nearby may impede the therapeutic interaction. An office removed from other work areas and/or with sufficient soundproofing is ideal. If necessary, try to hold sessions during times when nearby spaces are not in use.

Children with autism spectrum disorder or sensory issues may have a heightened sensitivity to sound and may find even moderate sounds disturbing or painful. Therapists using music should take special care not to overload a child's sensory system and introduce new sounds slowly. Macintyre (2015) notes that some educators allow children to listen to white noise with the intention of filtering out environmental stimuli that overstimulates them. Noise-cancelling headphones can also be useful for children who have difficulty tolerating everyday sounds. If a child uses such headphones, the therapist should follow the child's lead when using music and allow the child to decide when and whether to remove them.

We can now begin to look at techniques for how to use music when working with a child. The following sections provide an overview of activities that can be used in the therapy room.

LISTENING TO INSTRUMENTAL MUSIC AND SONGS

Listening to music with another person creates a shared experience. Whether sitting side by side or across a room, the music binds therapist and client together and brings them into a space of collective understanding. In assessing how music may be introduced into a session, the child or adolescent will offer immediate cues for how to proceed. Some children are naturally musical and may come into the room humming or speaking in a sing-song way. Others may enter wearing ear buds, listening to music already—instead of asking them to take them off you can start by asking what they are listening to, and what they feel about the music.

When planning to offer a music-listening experience to your client, you can use your phone, computer, or tablet to store songs. A Bluetooth speaker with good resonant sound is useful to have in the therapy room. Having two or three playlists of different kinds of songs is helpful in meeting the needs of the moment. If the child is energetic, having a series of songs that begin with a higher level of energy and then gradually become slower in tempo can lead the child into a calmer state. For very young children you may want to choose familiar songs, for example "The Wheels on the Bus," "The Itsy Bitsy Spider," and "Are You Sleeping?" The progression of these three songs moves from energetic and physical in nature, to a focus on singing, to becoming more relaxed and quiet.

With older children and adolescents, consider songs that are appropriate to chronological and developmental age, family dynamics, and culture. Many children will be hesitant to give a choice, so again you can have a playlist of songs at the ready. Children may choose something they like from the playlist; they may also choose something their parents listen to at home, such as The Beatles. Sometimes using your own set of preferred songs is a good tactic—develop one set that has a variety of styles on it that you can move through, including a classical piece (e.g., a Mozart piano sonata), blues song ("Nobody Knows When You're Down and Out"), folk ("Puff the Magic Dragon"), and contemporary (from *Billboard*'s Top 100 list). If you need help finding suitable songs, websites like www.theteachersguide.com have many resources for finding songs, printing lyrics, and watching videos of songs you would like to learn.

SINGING

It may happen that a child or teen you are treating is eager to sing—and wants you to sing along with him. Children often request to sing their favorite songs and derive great pleasure from singing them again and again. You do not need any special music or vocal training to join in singing. Some people are self-conscious about their vocal quality and ability to carry a tune. It is important to face any fears you might have regarding singing with others. When singing with children, keep in mind that you are not performing and that no one is judging you. If you see yourself as a participant rather than a performer, it will be easier to relax and focus on the song, not on yourself (Jalongo & Collins, 1985). The important thing for nonmusicians to remember is that children respond most when others show their enjoyment of singing. Try to find a balance between your voice and the child's voice—sing loud enough to be heard, but not loud enough to overpower the child. Instrumental accompaniment on piano or guitar is not necessary. Your voice is your most valuable musical instrument, and an in-tune voice is perfectly sufficient (Jalongo & Collins, 1985). Of course, you can always accompany on percussion instruments such as a drum or tambourine, or use body percussion: clapping hands, stamping feet, snapping fingers, or tapping on other parts of the body. Sharing your enthusiasm is more important than your level of musical skill, so do not be afraid to sing out! Gradually, your confidence will grow.

Children naturally move to music, so it is likely that your client will want to move as he sings. Movement can be anything from gentle swaying to the beat to energetic dancing around the room. Be prepared to join in. If you feel inhibited about moving to music, practice on your own moving to different kinds of music. Put on some of your favorite music and begin by swaying and moving your arms. Relax, breathe, and allow your body to move naturally to the rhythms of the song. If you feel awkward, take a scarf and wave it in time to the music. As you become more comfortable doing this, make larger and larger movements, until you are moving back and forth in an easy, fluid manner.

If you do not know a song that your client asks for, you can tell the child that you will learn it or bring it in for the next session. It is usually easy to find a song on the Internet; there are websites available that you can use to search for lyrics, like *www.chordie.com* and *www.lyrics.com*, and you can listen to countless songs on *www.youtube.com*. Listen to the song several times and then try singing along with the recording until you feel confident that you have learned the melody and words. Again, work within your comfort level. Sometimes not being as musical as your client can be a confidence builder for him; there are times to support and celebrate a client's musicality.

WORKING WITH SONG LYRICS

Well-known songs can be used creatively in the therapy room. The child can play along with the pulse of the song or tap the rhythm of the words and melody (known as the melodic rhythm), or talk about the words. Reading lyrics aloud and talking about their relevance to a client's life can provide a useful, indirect means of addressing sensitive issues. Changing the lyrics of songs with active input from your client can also be a powerful tool.

Another way of working with lyrics is to build vocabulary and concepts with word substitution songs. This is especially useful when working with children with language delays. For example, most people know "Old MacDonald Had a Farm," where the children fill in the names of animals and their respective sounds. There are songs about body parts, such as Woody Guthrie's "Put Your Finger in the Air," where the child names a body part to put his finger on and creates a corresponding rhyme. Songs can teach or reinforce various concepts. Perhaps the most widely known is the "The ABC Song"; other examples include songs about the body ("Head, Shoulders, Knees and Toes"), counting songs ("Five Little Monkeys"), songs about daily living skills ("Here We Go 'Round the Mulberry Bush"), and countless more. (See Chapter 7 for more detail about using lyrics to facilitate language development.)

Finding songs your client prefers, or drawing upon your own memory of favorite childhood songs if the client is hesitant or unwilling to choose, is a good starting point for working with song lyrics. Adding lyrics that are personalized to the child, whether about his actions, mood, or words, creates a whole new song that is uniquely his. Seven-year-old Sam came into the therapy room exuberantly stating, "I'm here!" Meeting his energy, I (L. E. B.) smiled and started singing, to the tune of "If You're Happy and You Know It," "When Sam is in the room he says 'I'm here!' [I'm here!]." This song became a regular part of our greeting in subsequent sessions.

If a child enters the room with a shy demeanor or avoiding eye contact, you may want to acknowledge and support this reticence in the context of a song. For example, adapting the song "Where Is Thumbkin?" yields many possibilities for meaning and personal connection. Singing "Where is Natalie, where is Natalie?" while she hides in the room, then "There she is! There she is!" when you 'find' her, is a cogent means to enact a healthy engagement in a fun, playful, and, for the child, exciting way. You can then "hide" and allow Natalie to sing and find you. In both of the examples above, the therapist takes her cues from how the child presents herself: with high or low energy? With words and eye contact? By matching this energy and level of interaction and putting it into a familiar song, you impart the message that you are ready to meet the child in whatever mood he is in.

Taking a familiar song and studying the lyrics in a meaningful way can have several benefits: trust is increased between client and therapist; cognitive skills can be worked on in a satisfying and unintimidating fashion; communication is fostered by sharing thoughts and ideas about lyrics; and personal histories can be shared in a nonintrusive manner.

When listening to a song and focusing on the lyrics, we suggest allowing some time for silence before jumping in with a comment or question. The silence allows space for thoughts and feelings to surface.

Wait to see if the child spontaneously makes a comment. Carefully observe the child's facial expression and body language—these will give you clues about how he is feeling—without staring directly at him. It is best to look in a neutral place, so the child does not feel pressured to respond before he is ready.

The therapist has the choice whether to process the experience verbally, or to simply sit quietly with the feelings in the room. For clinicians not used to using music, waiting to comment on the experience can be uncomfortable at first, but doing so sets a precedent of allowing time for the child to absorb the lyrics and to respond first. If you decide to open a verbal discussion, try to avoid asking direct questions that might be perceived as intimidating or leading. As will be discussed in Chapter 3, keep comments objective and specific. It is often useful to begin a phrase with "I wonder . . ." followed by a comment that may, in fact, imply a question without asking it directly. The child is free to respond, or he can choose not to respond—either way, the message is that it is okay. Here are some examples:

- "I wonder if that song reminded you of something." [connecting an observed emotional response to the song]
- "I noticed that when the music got loud and fast, you put your head down. I wonder what you were feeling at that moment." [gently inquiring about an observed response]
- "I noticed that when the singer sang about wanting to go home, you looked sad. I wonder if that is what you were feeling." [connecting possible emotional response to an issue being worked on]

When working with older children, giving them the opportunity to choose songs and make up new lyrics is empowering and creatively fulfilling. The child suggests new phrases that fit the melody and rhythm of the song. Taking the chorus and changing the words based on your client's experiences is a simple approach to creating meaningful new lyrics as shown in the vignette below.

VIGNETTE

Sheri was a 12-year-old girl who attended middle school in a predominantly middle-class neighborhood. She was being seen by Gwen, a school counselor, for failing grades. The first session was spent chatting and with Gwen getting to know Sheri. Nothing dramatic was revealed, though Sheri did acknowledge she was worried about her grades. She said she did not know what had changed or why school was suddenly so hard. She had gone through a battery of tests that did not reveal any changes in cognition or attention span. As soon as she walked into Gwen's office for the second session she started crying. Gwen offered support and tissues and waited until Sheri had calmed down before asking her what was going on. Sheri pulled herself together and defiantly said, "Nothing." She refused to say what was bothering her and started to get angry over being asked: "It's none of your business!" she practically shouted.

Gwen took a minute to gather her thoughts. She knew if she pushed Sheri she risked alienating her and that she might not come back. She asked Sheri if she could put on a song they could listen to, and when Sheri nodded her head in agreement, Gwen gave her a choice between "Confident" by Demi Lovato and "Fight Song" by Rachel Platten. Sheri, without looking up, said "Fight Song." Gwen played the song using her phone and a Bluetooth speaker, at a moderate level. When it finished she asked Sheri if she would like to hear it again, this time a little louder. Sheri agreed again, this time with a hint of a smile. Gwen turned the volume up a bit and noticed that they both started bobbing their heads and tapping their feet in time to the music. She felt this synchrony opened a door to communication, and so when the song ended she asked Sheri, "What do you think of the song?" Sheri replied, "I dunno, it's just a really good song." Gwen felt unsure of where to go next but felt inspired to say, "In the song, fighting is a good thing, isn't it? It says she's going to stay strong, even when life gets tough. Do you agree?" Sheri was silent for few seconds, then responded, "Yeah. Keep fighting, keep going, even when it all sucks. I think that's cool." Gwen nodded her head, agreeing, and waited a minute before speaking again. When she did, she said, "I'd like to read those lyrics. Would you?" Sheri said yes, and Gwen went to her computer and printed two copies.

First, they read the lyrics silently, then Gwen played the song again while they sang along. Sheri's voice got stronger with each verse and by the end of the song she was making sporadic eye contact with Gwen and smiling. When the song ended they broke into spontaneous laughter, sharing the moment of connection. Gwen suggested they write some of their own lyrics at the next session, and Sheri replied, "Yeah, that'd be cool." In their next session they rewrote some of the lyrics to the chorus, with Sheri offering "This is my fight song, my stand up and do it song" as a suggestion. Gwen noticed that Sheri was able to think of imaginative lines that fit the melodic contour of the song.

Over the course of the next two sessions they continued to work on changing the lyrics of the song. Sheri became more confident, disagreeing with Gwen when she thought a line should be written a different way, and even suggesting she sing it alone once they finished. The final version contained some lyrics centered on the girl protagonist feeling strong, even when people made fun of her clothes or how she talked. Gwen noted that when Sheri sang this part of the song her voice became even clearer and stronger. After singing the song, the conversation turned to how Sheri was doing in school. She spoke in a confident voice, even while sharing that her mom did not have the money to get her new clothes and that she sometimes felt embarrassed by how she dressed.

After getting Sheri's permission, Gwen shared this information with Sheri's teacher who had been wondering why Sheri seemed so withdrawn. He said he would be more alert to Sheri's state of mind and, over the next few weeks, Sheri's grades began to climb. She carried herself differently, standing taller than she had before, and was able to make eye contact more easily. Gwen believed that their work on the song helped Sheri develop confidence while letting Gwen know what was bothering her. She thought there might be more to Sheri's story, but that there was time for them to work on any other issues that might arise.

USING MUSICAL INSTRUMENTS

There are two basic rules when using instruments with clients: no one gets hurt and no instruments get damaged. This may seem obvious, yet instilling a sense of respect for the instruments is a mirror for respecting the therapeutic process. For example, when first using an instrument with a client, we recommend you become more formal in your movements, slow down a bit, and handle instruments gently. Children notice and respond to this type of honoring; it becomes natural to them for instruments to be handled with a sense of reverence.

When introducing instruments to the therapy setting, consider your comfort level and your musical abilities. If you are hesitant to play a drum, you may not want to include drums in your practice. Your client may sense your unease and either exhibit hesitancy or try to dominate the experience by playing loudly and uncontrollably. Identify the instruments you are comfortable with and use those. Similarly, the child needs to feel comfortable playing, although he may also benefit from encountering new experiences and challenges. Appendix A itemizes and describes the many instruments that can be used with children.

Introduce instruments one at a time and demonstrate how to play them and the sounds they produce. There might be more than one way; for instance, a tambourine can be shaken in the air, tapped with a hand, or tapped on various parts of the body. Offer the instrument to the child to explore. Children may find unique ways to play, and it is important to nurture their creativity while at the same time using the instrument as it was intended. Instruments should be used functionally to create sound. If the child mishandles the instrument in a way that can be destructive, explain that a mallet is for tapping, not for throwing or banging; maracas are for shaking, not for spinning on the floor.

You may also opt to start by having a few instruments in the room and allowing the child to explore them freely. Many children are curious and naturally drawn to particular instruments and want to investigate how to play them. We recommend having two small drums with mallets, three or four resonator bells from a given key (e.g., C, E, and G bars for the key of C), and three or four egg shakers. This collection gives the child a choice and gives you the leeway to choose either a similar instrument or a contrasting one.

Either the therapist or the child can initiate instrumental playing. The therapist can begin and invite the child to choose an instrument and join in. Be careful not to overwhelm the child with too many choices. Alternatively, the child can choose an instrument and initiate playing. Whether you join in and play along depends on the child and his needs. You can ask "May I play with you?" and see how the child responds. Some children like to play alone and hear more clearly what they are doing. We recommend that you have duplicates of some of the instruments—two drums, two tambourines, two similar melodic instruments—so that you can engage in parallel play.

Another option is to have the child play along to recorded music (e.g., playing a drum to rhythmic music such as a rock song or a march). The music can be chosen by either the therapist or the child. Web applications like Spotify, Pandora, or Google Music have capabilities to find existing playlists for children, or for you to create your own as you discover musical selections you think will be useful in the clinical setting.

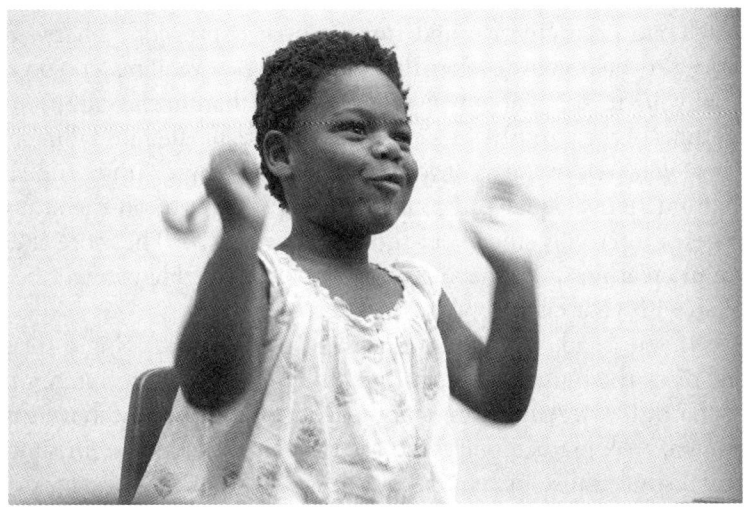

Girl playing xylimba

IMPROVISATION

In improvisation, we use the elements of music—rhythm, melody, harmony, dynamics, timbre, and form—to create something new to meet the needs of the client. Improvising with children does not require sophisticated musical knowledge or training. It does require a willingness to join in musical experimentation and to listen with sensitivity to what the child is trying to communicate. When engaging in improvisation, the therapist must try to lose any self-consciousness or judgment about "performance" or sounding "good," and instead listen to what the child is trying to express. The goal is not to make "pretty" or aesthetically pleasing music (though this may happen), but rather to create something that is an authentic expression of the child's feeling. The therapist can play an instrument or vocalize simultaneously with the child, establish a game of musical turn-taking, or simply serve as a witness to let the child know that someone is listening. It is important to remember to leave space, in the form of pauses or silences, for the child's spontaneous expressions. The therapist must also resist the urge to lead the child too much, instead allowing the child's experience to unfold organically.

Children love to experiment with sounds and to make up their own songs—this is one form of improvisation. Using syllables or nonsense words can be a creative and fun personal expression. There are techniques to help you develop this skill. Practice making up songs about what you are doing at any given moment. When in the car, listen to the rhythms of the windshield wipers and sing about the rain falling or about where you are driving to. If you are riding a subway or train, tune into the rhythmic movements and sounds and tap them out on the seat or your knee, or internally sing about the scenery going by. The more at ease you are in creating spontaneous songs, the more quickly you will be able to do so with your clients.

If you decide to improvise with instruments, keeping a steady beat organizes the music and helps the child play in a more intentional, less haphazard way. All children, and particularly those who have suffered a trauma, seek predictability and safety, so it is best to begin simply. Setting a stable pulse or tempo on a drum or other instrument, or repeating two alternating notes either sung or played on a pitched instrument such as a xylophone or piano, can create a grounding experience that provides needed safety and familiarity. External rhythm brings internal order, and a child can find security in consistency and repetitions of rhythmic phrases. You can give your client a frame drum and mallet, and say, "Why don't you start?" If the child starts beating very energetically, you can briefly match this and then create a strong steady beat that the child can play over. If the child starts by playing tentatively, with only a few, scattered, soft beats, you can briefly match his way of playing and initiate a steady, soft beat for the child to play with. Having a clear tonal center (the key of the music) provides another means of creating stability, and once this is established you can begin to improvise off of it.

When listening to a child play music, there are many considerations to keep in mind. Begin by simply listening and noting how the child is playing and how the music sounds. Questions you might ask yourself include:

- What is the quality of the music? Does it sound peaceful or dramatic?
- Does the playing tend to be loud/soft, fast/slow?
- What is the child's body language communicating? For example, if he is playing loudly, is he smiling, or does he look angry? Does his body seem tense or relaxed? Is he using small or large movements?

- Does the child's playing stay the same over time, or does it change? Can he play both fast and slow, both loud and soft? Rigidity in playing suggests rigidity in thinking and in ways of interacting in the world. One goal could be to increase flexibility so that he is better able to respond to life situations and engage in mutual and satisfying interactions with others.
- Does he initiate changes or follow changes—or both? Communication is a two-way street—sometimes we speak, sometimes we listen. Sometimes we lead, sometimes we follow. Children can practice this back-and-forth in a musical context. A child who insists upon leading may need to be encouraged to listen. A child who prefers to follow can be encouraged to initiate.

Careful observation will reveal vital information about how the child feels about himself and the world. It is important to trust your instincts here, yet also, if possible, check your perceptions with the client. What sounds loud or angry to one person may sound determined or emphatic to another. Visual cues are important to note as well. A child playing loudly and aggressively looks qualitatively different from a child playing loudly and exuberantly, while a child playing anxiously in a fast tempo looks different from a child playing happily in a fast tempo. We may not know the root of the child's aggression or anxiety, but we can be fairly certain of how he is feeling in that moment.

While music is ordered and organized by rhythm and other elements, improvisation by its very nature is unpredictable, since we do not know exactly what is going to happen next. Within this apparent contradiction lies the beauty of musical improvisation, as it can contain both predictability and ambiguity at the same time (Turry, 2002). A child can be gently guided toward a greater tolerance of uncertainty within an emotionally safe musical experience.

The experience of making music freely can be satisfying and empowering. When improvising, the child is given the opportunity to make many decisions regarding use of voice or instrument: how fast or slow, loud or soft the music should be, whether he will add vocal sounds or words and what these might be. Being able to lead the music builds a child's confidence and encourages him to take future risks in the service of greater openness and health. Having a sense of partnership in the creation of the music helps children to overcome poor self-image or a lack of confidence.

WORKING WITH THE FORM AND STRUCTURE OF MUSIC

Music imparts experiences of form and order, from the simple to the highly complex. The structure of music, with its rhythms and tempo, provides stability and organization. These experiences are fundamental not only to music, but to life in general (Nordoff & Robbins, 2007). We all rely on routine and the comfort of anticipating certain events in our daily lives—otherwise, life would be confusing or even incomprehensible. This is the feeling some children experience when, due to internal or external causes, they are not able to organize their own behavior, thoughts, or emotions. Music demands time-ordered behavior (Sears, 1968), and children feel secure when listening to or playing within a musical structure. The organization inherent in music leads to experience in self-organization, which in turn leads to self-expression. Music exists only in time—this necessitates moment-to-moment commitment by the individual. The therapist can adjust to the client's responses to meet changing needs in the moment (Sears, 1968).

At the heart of verbal and social interactions is a rhythmic exchange in the form of question–answer or a call-and-response that is nonverbal, yet implicitly understood. Most human interactions can be reduced to sounds, rhythms, and/or movements that do not require words; we can understand much of what someone is communicating just by listening to the tone and inflections behind the words. By deemphasizing the words and instead relying on rhythmically driven music, a therapist can "cultivate interpersonal rhythms" (Porges, 2011, xvi) with even the most aggressive or remote child.

A child with impulse control issues may find it difficult to control or stop certain behaviors. However, engaging in a song with clear starts and stops affords an opportunity to initiate and terminate actions in a pleasurable way. A song such as "This Old Man" can be adapted so that after singing the number of a verse ("he played two"), the child plays a tone bar two times and then stops before singing the rest of the phrase. This gives him the experience of starting and stopping on time that makes the song sound complete. It gives him an internal sense of control and satisfaction. In fact, the most basic musical form is sound versus no sound, or sound versus silence. When children grasp this form, they delight in being able to control the sounds that they and others produce by cueing when to play and when to stop; this aids in the development of impulse control.

Adding layers of complexity to a song can be helpful in many ways: it can be used to improve sequencing skills, enhance attention, foster positive interactions, and increase pride of accomplishment. Taking the previous example of "This Old Man," a therapist may sing through the song with a child in a session, and in the next session bring in a hand drum. For every number in a verse, the child plays the drum for the specific number of times, increasing from 1 to 10. If this experience is successful, the therapist can bring in two instruments the next time and have the child alternate between the two for each of the numbers. Building further on that, the therapist could increase the number of instruments to 10 and, in the moment, indicate which instrument the child should play for any given number. There are of course many variations possible here, and you can return to previous reenactments of the song if the child struggles with an added level of complexity.

A stable harmonic form, such as a repeated chord progression on guitar, is another way to provide structure. Participating in antiphonal (call and response) repeating of patterns helps create and sustain two-way communication; this can be particularly helpful for children who find it challenging to interact with others. Imitating rhythmic patterns requires the child to listen to a pattern before beating it, process the perceived information, and plan and produce a motor response. Success requires focus and leads to feelings of competence. Adding musical punctuation at the ends of phrases, such as a striking a triangle at the end of a drum pattern or a line of a song, helps to focus a child's attention and give purpose to his playing.

Making music is fun, and when a child plays his part well it sounds and feels enjoyable. Working with the form and structure of music provides many opportunities for mastery. It increases confidence and strengthens the child's ability to interact with the therapist and, in turn, with others in his life.

WORKING WITH IMAGERY AND THEMES

Music lends itself to use with imagery and the development of themes. Listening to music can evoke images of nature, experiences, places, people, as well as fantasy. Images evoked by music are intensely personal. For example, when hearing march-like music in a strong, steady tempo, one child might picture a festival with people dancing, while another child might conjure up images of war and tragedy. Thus, music can be thought of as a blank slate upon which each listener projects his own thoughts and writes his own story, like a Rorschach inkblot. What we hear in music tells us a great deal about ourselves—our perceptions, personality, and emotions.

Discussing the imagery inspired by music can illuminate unconscious thoughts and feelings that are brought to the surface. To elicit a conversation, the therapist needs to ask open-ended questions that encourage the child to articulate his experience, such as:

- "What pictures did you see in your mind when you were listening?"
- "Sometimes music takes us on a journey. Did you imagine that you traveled somewhere while you were listening?"

Sometimes a child comes into a session with a strong emotion that lends itself to creating imagery. This is an opportunity for you to be creative—when choosing an image to explore, we are limited only by our imagination. Perhaps the child is feeling angry and is having difficulty expressing his anger. One idea is to tell a story in music about a thunderstorm. Together with the child you can choose various instruments to depict different parts of the storm (possible suggestions are in parentheses below). Take your time and allow the child to fully explore each instrument and contribute verbally to the narrative. The story starts with dark clouds rolling in (sand blocks, guiro), followed by gentle raindrops (wood blocks, xylophone). The wind begins to pick up (wind chimes, reed horns) and the rainfall becomes heavy (ocean drum, bongos). Suddenly there is lightning and thunder (drum rolls, hand cymbals), getting louder and louder. After it reaches a climax, the storm begins to die down; the intensity of the rain lessens, and eventually slows and stops (repeat instruments previously used or add others). Finally, the sun comes out (jingle or pitched bells) and the storm has passed. This kind of activity can provide a cathartic experience for a child: he has had an opportunity to express his anger through powerful sound making, and then is returned to a more calm and regulated state. The musical storm has allowed him to take a symbolic emotional journey with you.

Often, a child will introduce into the therapy session some area of interest to him, be it superheroes, trains, numbers, baseball, or virtually anything else. When trying to engage a child, it is common practice to begin with the child's own interests rather than to impose your own agenda. So, the question is, how do you translate a child's topic of interest into sound? One way is to create a story based on the theme and to add instruments, as in the example of the thunderstorm above. In creating a baseball theme, you might ask, "What instrument sounds like the crack of a bat? What does it sound like when a batter hits a home run and the crowd roars?" When exploring a superhero theme, you might ask, "What instrument do you think Superman would want to play?" Once that is decided, you can ask, "How would he play it?" You can begin the narration, setting the scene and talking about what Superman might be saying through the music, and then invite the child's contribution with statements such as "I wonder what happens next." It is best to avoid asking too many direct questions, as the child might feel like he is being interrogated or put on the spot.

Another strategy is to create a chant or song based on a theme, using the child's own words as a starting point. You can elaborate on the theme by adding your own words and ideas, always being mindful of the child's response of acceptance or rejection. The goal is to help him develop his ideas in the context of a shared, interactive experience. Although you can allow the child to lead, there are times when you will likely take a supportive role and times when you might lead the child into new territory. Brian, a 7-year-old child, came into therapy exhibiting signs of anxiety because he was being bullied at school. His therapist, William, felt that focusing on his name could be an empowering process. Once he felt a rapport had been established, he engaged Brian in a light-hearted exploration of what their names sounded like. They started by sounding out Brian's name and elongating the syllables, taking turns with each name, and then adding some vocal sound effects, for example, saying "Briiiiii-AN!" Before long they were laughing together at the sounds they were making. William shifted the play into chanting each of their names in a strong rhythm. This became something Brian enjoyed doing, and they started each session chanting his name, each time trying out new expressions and ways of sounding out the syllables.

MUSIC IN GROUP WORK

Music can enhance the processes of developing trust and cohesion in a group setting. Playing and listening to music together establishes common ground and creates healthy boundaries: one child's preferences will be different from another child's. Engaging in someone else's preferred style of music in a respectful manner can create an atmosphere of comradery. The therapist needs to be clear in setting boundaries and ground rules for respecting each other's choices.

Song writing in groups can build group trust and cohesion. A topic may emerge organically from a group discussion or from one group member, or the therapist can initiate a topic she feels has relevance for the clients. Each group member is asked to contribute to the lyrics, which can be chanted or put to a simple melody. A simple accompaniment of two alternating chords, or two large tone bars, can provide stability yet create an open feeling of possibility. The words can be written down or the song recorded to become a part of the group's unique repertoire. Clients may learn that others share their concerns, and that they are not alone. Or, they may realize that group members have different perspectives and that they cannot assume others think or feel the same way they do. Any conflicts that arise due to differences in how a song should sound, or what words to insert, can, with the guidance of the therapist, be negotiated and resolved through compromise. By keeping the focus on the song, the therapist can work with conflict so that it does not become personal. These experiences are invaluable in building acceptance, understanding, cooperation, and empathy.

Musical dramas are another creative avenue for group exploration; these can be developed from known stories or improvised. There are many childhood stories that address issues important to children: conquering fears, dealing with family and all its permutations, getting along with others, staying true to one's own self, balancing dependence versus independence, coping with difficult life circumstances, and more. Think about the issues your clients are working on and if you know a story with a relevant theme. For example, children who are timid or perhaps bullied may relate to the story of "The Three Billy Goats Gruff." In this tale, the billy goats must work together to outsmart a threatening ogre. In Nordoff and Robbins's adaptation of the Grimm fairy tale "Fair Katrinelje and Pif-Paf-Poltrie" (1961, see Chapter 5), Pif's hard work "putting his house in order" ultimately leads to a good life with satisfying relationships. After choosing a story, discuss with your clients the different instruments that might represent the characters or other elements in the story, and how the story could be brought to life. Props, staging, writing dialogue, and learning it can all be part of this collaborative experience.

SUMMARY

This chapter presented the basic considerations and techniques for getting started in using music therapeutically with children. It provided specific guidelines for setting up an office that is conducive to the use of music as well as techniques such as listening, singing, and improvisation that can be implemented by professionals who are not necessarily trained or proficient in music. The next chapter takes this one step further and shows how music can be integrated with other forms of practice to achieve therapeutic goals.

RECOMMENDATIONS FOR PRACTICE

There are many ways music can be introduced into therapy. What follows here are suggestions for how a therapist might create music experiences in individual sessions and in groups. These are flexible and adaptable, for ideas proposed for individual work may also be suited for group work and vice versa.

Working with Clients Individually

Question and Answer and Call and Response

- The therapist and the child both choose an instrument and sit facing each other. Give instructions that in this musical activity one of you will be asking a question, but not using words, and the other person will be answering by using his instrument.
- Go back and forth a few times, and if your client can engage verbally, ask what it was like to hear a question and an answer in music—was it similar to using words? What was different? Could you tell what the question might be?
- Switch roles and repeat.

Stop and Go

- The therapist controls the start and stop of a piece of recorded music and has the child play when the music starts, and stop when the music stops.

- Another level of structure for this is to move the volume up and down, with the express instruction that the child is to follow the dynamic changes and mirror them in his play.
- As this activity becomes familiar, the child can take a turn controlling the music starting and stopping, and its volume.

Ostinato

An ostinato is a short, repeated musical phrase or rhythm. Ostinati are often used in jazz or rock music, where they may be referred to as a riff or vamp; they are also common in classical music.

- An ostinato can be as simple as two alternating tones, for example, going back and forth between two chime bars a fifth apart (e.g., D and the A above it) or a fourth apart (e.g., G and the C above it).
- When played in a moderately slow tempo, this simple pattern provides a stable accompaniment and serves as a foundation for other music played or sung over it.
- An ostinato can also be a short rhythmic pattern played on a drum or other percussion instrument.

Identifying a Theme (Weather, Favorite Food, Mood, Favorite Place) and Creating a Short Rhythmic Chant

- Create the chant using the syllables of a few relevant words.
- Focus on the rhythm of the word or phrase and play it on a small drum.
- Once you begin repeating it, it becomes an ostinato pattern that your client can play off of, either vocally or instrumentally. For example, if you choose "the ocean" as a theme, you would beat a steady pattern of *the o-cean* [pause]; *the o-cean* [pause]; your client could play another drum over your ostinato and improvise other rhythms, or could rhythmically add his own ideas of what he likes about being at the ocean, for example, *the wa-ter* [pause] *is blue* [pause], *the wa-ter* [pause] *is blue* [pause].
- Switch roles, so your client is playing the ostinato and you are improvising words or rhythms. This role reversal can be empowering for children in therapy.

- If the child sustains loud playing, preventing you from being heard, or attempts to stop you from playing, you can end the music by stating "And now it's time to stop!" and gathering the instruments to put away.

Working with Groups

- Emphasis can be placed upon taking individual turns within the group context, or on having the entire group play together with varying levels of structure and therapist oversight.
- Children take individual turns to go up and play a djembe or floor drum that is set in the middle of the group while the rest of the members play a steady beat on hand drums. The leader can cue those playing hand drums to play more quietly to better hear the soloist.
- *Stations:* Place instruments in different parts of the room so that the children are free to move around and explore. The therapist can unify the experience by keeping a steady beat on a drum, or the children can play along to recorded music.
- Pass a rhythm around a circle by chanting, clapping, or tapping on a hand drum. One approach to begin is to use the children's names: chant and/or tap the rhythmic patterns of names by using the number of syllables and the accents in a rhythmic manner; for example, three beats and a rest for LAU-ra BEER (rest), LAU-ra BEER (rest), and so on; or five beats—two eighth notes and three quarter notes—for [JAC-que]-line BIRN-baum, [JAC-que]-line BIRN-baum (repeat) (see Figure 2.1).

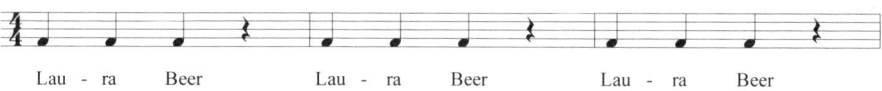

Lau - ra   Beer   Lau - ra   Beer   Lau - ra   Beer

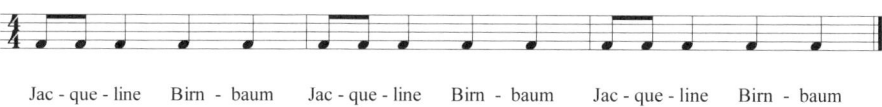

Jac - que - line   Birn - baum   Jac - que - line   Birn - baum   Jac - que - line   Birn - baum

FIGURE 2.1. Rhythm example

APPENDIX 2.1. SUGGESTED INSTRUMENTS AND EQUIPMENT

There are many considerations to keep in mind when selecting instruments to use with children. Toy companies make colorful and attractive sound-making toys that may look like small versions of real instruments like plastic guitars, metal xylophones, and others. However, it is most important to pay attention to the quality of the sound that is produced. No matter how alluring it may look, a toy that makes an unpleasant sound will soon lose its appeal. Like adults, children are attracted to aesthetically pleasing sounds. We recommend choosing real, not toy, instruments—it is worth the investment. Well-made instruments are made to withstand children's often forceful playing. Still, over time they may wear out or become damaged. All instruments must be kept in good repair, and fixed or replaced if broken or not working properly.

Many instruments can be adapted to suit the individual needs of your clients. For example, if a child is sensitive to loud sounds, putting strips of tape on the bottom of a cymbal will dampen the sound. There are many different types of mallets available; soft mallets may be good for children who tend to play strongly, while harder mallets will allow children who play softly to produce more sound.

Instruments we find particularly useful are listed below. One caution we offer is to only have instruments in the room you are comfortable playing yourself. For example, if you are not a pianist or guitarist, do not have these instruments in the treatment room, as children will naturally be drawn to playing them and not having proper support in their explorations of the instruments may only frustrate them. You can go to a local music store and experiment with different instruments and see if they fit your needs; employees at these stores can make recommendations as well. Avoid drums that have patterns, shapes, or colors on them as these can be distracting or even disturbing to clients with sensory processing issues.

- Drums: These vary by size and timbre:
  - Conga: a tall, narrow drum originally from Cuba, played with the hands.
  - Bongos: a pair of small, connected drums played with the hands.
  - Frame drum: a drum that has a drumhead width greater than its depth, played with the hands or a mallet.
  - Paddle drum: a frame drum mounted on a racquet handle, played with a mallet.
  - Buffalo drum: similar to a frame drum, but with a rope handle on the underside; inspired by native American cultures; played with the hands or a mallet.

- Djembe: a rope-tuned, skin covered drum originally from West Africa, played with the hands.
    - Tubano: a tall, cylindrical drum with sturdy feet, played with the hands.
    - Ocean drum: a double-sided frame drum containing metal beads, played by shaking or gently tilting it as the beads roll against the drum head to create a sound like the ocean.
- A variety of sticks and mallets of different lengths and made of different materials (rubber, yarn, wood, felt, or other materials).
- Other percussion instruments:
    - Durable plastic or wood maracas.
    - Tambourine.
    - Egg shakers.
    - Cluster bells, hand-held sleigh bells, or other bells for shaking.
    - Cabasa: a Latin percussion instrument made of loops of steel ball chain around a wide cylinder with a handle.
    - Woodblock and stick.
    - Sand blocks.
    - Pair of rhythm sticks (usually one smooth and one ridged) or claves (cylindrical hardwood sticks).
    - Guiro with striker: a notched, hollowed-out gourd played by rubbing a stick or scraper along the notches.
    - Triangle and striker.
    - Hand cymbals.
- Melodic instruments allow a child to create melodies:
    - Xylophone or xylimba. A xylimba is a wooden instrument similar to a xylophone; the difference is that each bar is tied on and cannot be taken off.
    - Metallophone: A metallophone is similar to a xylophone except that the bars are made of metal instead of wood.
    - Glockenspiel: a small metallophone, higher in pitch.
    - Resonator bells (also known as chime bars or tone bars): tuned metal bars with each bar mounted on its own wooden or plastic resonant box; played with a mallet.
    - Desk bells—these colorful bells are easy to play by tapping them on the top.
- Reed horn: a small metal horn that holds a single reed and produces one tone, played by blowing into the mouthpiece. Some are designed so that you can change the reed and thus change the tone. They must be sanitized after

each use with a cleanser such as Sterisol, a germicide designed for cleaning mouthpieces.
- Keyboard or piano (if the therapist knows how to play).
- String instruments:
    - Guitar–full-size, ½ size, and/or ¼ size (if the therapist knows how to play).
    - Small harp or zither: played by strumming or plucking the strings.
    - Autoharp: played by strumming and pushing buttons to create chords.
    - Ukulele: generally played by strumming (if the therapist knows how to play).
- Device with Internet access for listening to songs requested by clients, such as an iPad; access to quality speakers.

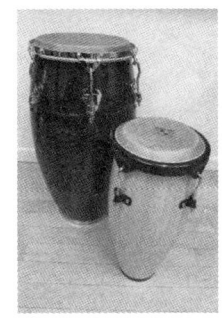 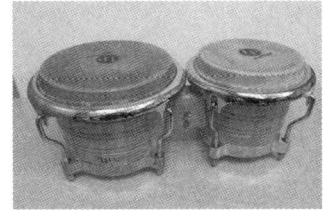

Conga drums   Bongos

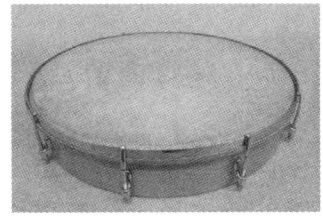 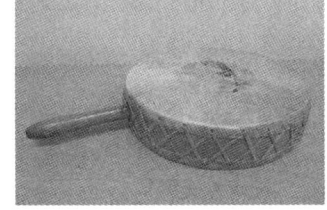

Frame drum   Paddle drum

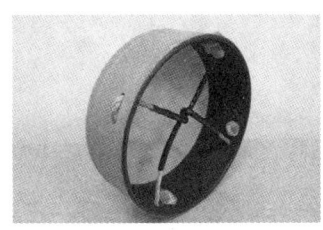 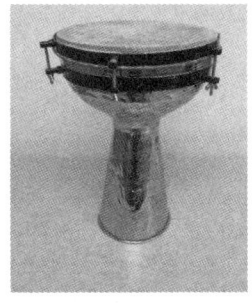

Buffalo drum   Djembe

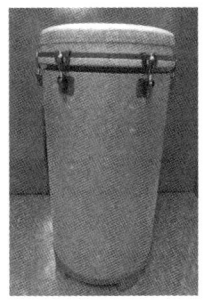 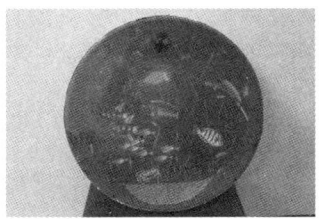

Tubano   Ocean drum

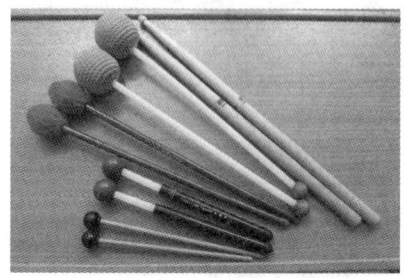 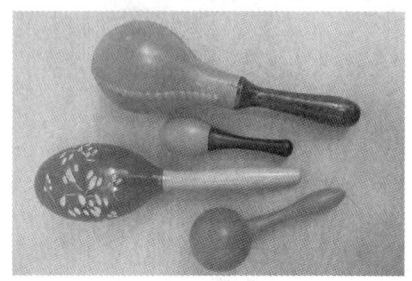

Sticks and mallets   Maracas

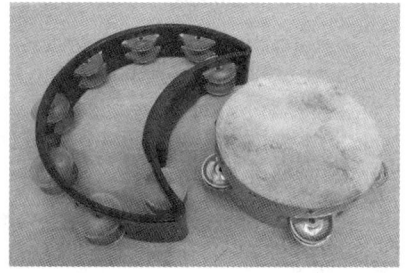 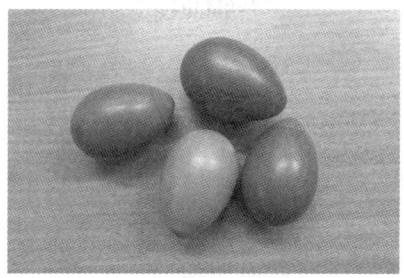

Tambourines   Egg shakers

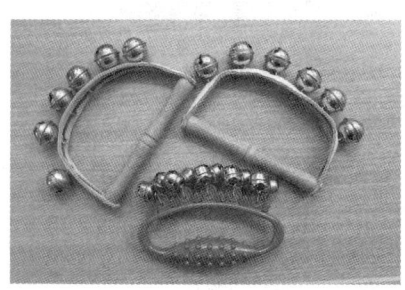 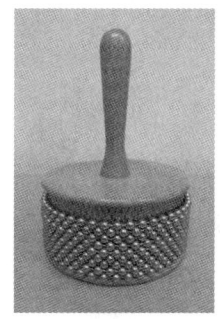

Cluster bells   Cabasa

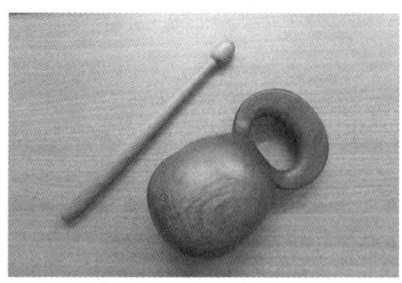 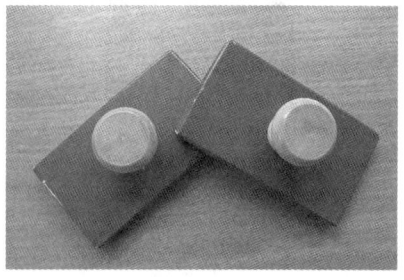

Woodblock   Sand blocks

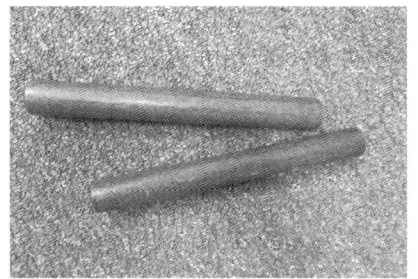

Claves

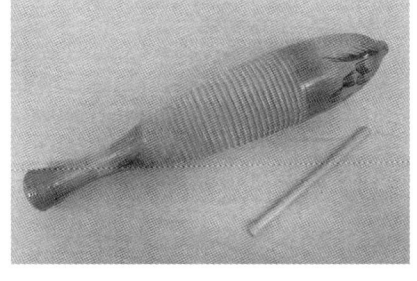

Guiro

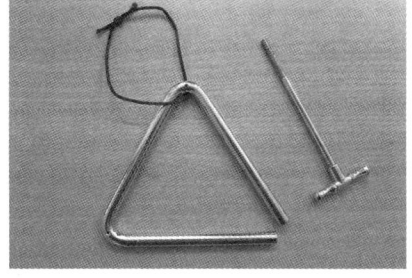

Triangle and striker

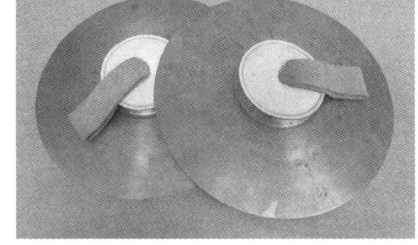

Hand cymbals

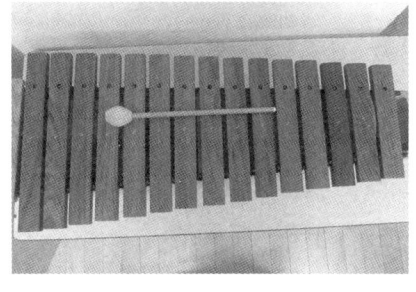

Xylophone

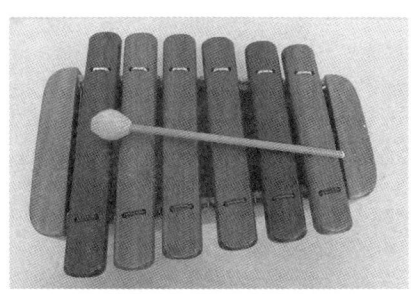

Xylimba

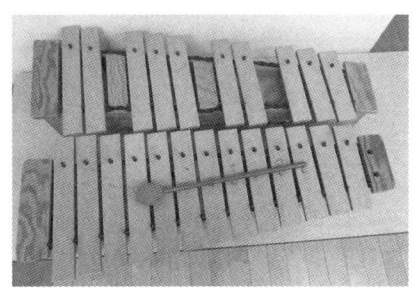

Metallophone

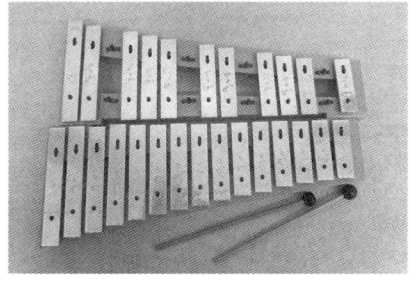

Glockenspiel

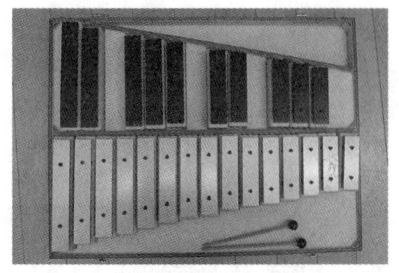
Resonator bells

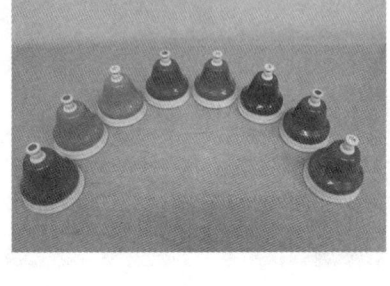
Desk bells

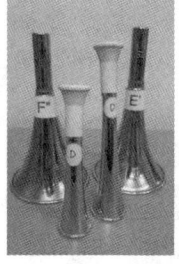
Reed horns

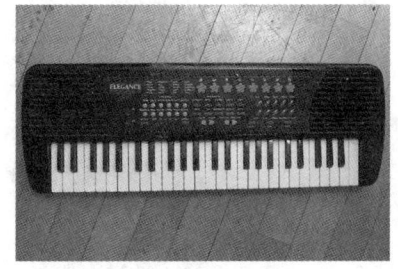
Keyboard

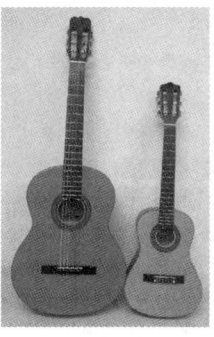
Guitars

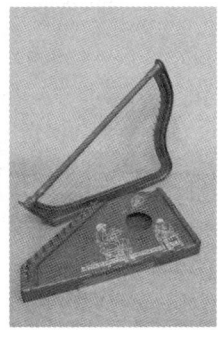
Harp and zither

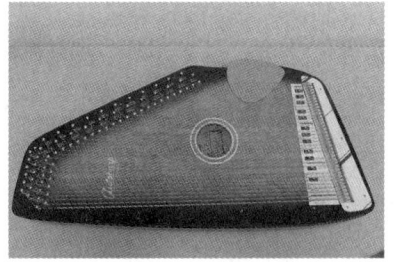
Autoharp

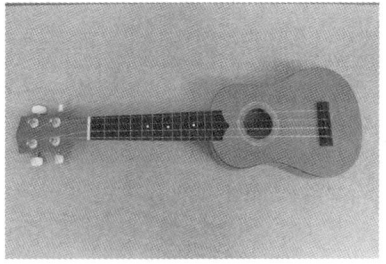
Ukulele

CHAPTER 3

Working with Music as an Agent of Change

>Where words fail, music speaks.
>—HANS CHRISTIAN ANDERSEN
>(as cited in Galowitz, 2001, p. 5)

Bringing music into the therapy room can build trust, help clients feel accepted, and create room for growth and change. Musical interventions intrinsically promote engagement and generate feelings of accomplishment so that children can reshape their behaviors and patterns of communication. Creating these music-oriented experiences within an environment of success requires a unique set of skills. The emphasis of this chapter is on helping the clinician to construct a setting in which the child feels supported and able to be successful when engaged in music making or listening.

There is inherent value in the anticipation of music, which is a form of musical cognition related to recognition and memory. Think about the pleasure and satisfaction we get from hearing music that we are familiar with: people know the lyrics to the songs of their favorite performers and sing along at their concerts; we sing the same holiday songs year after year. This familiarity gives us a sense that we know who we are and where we belong, and connects us to our families and communities in a profound way.

A child brings to therapy his full musical history. Perhaps music was sung in the home—parents singing lullabies to help children go to sleep, for example—or perhaps not. Knowing whether the parents or guardians play any instruments in the home and what they like to listen to is also valuable information, for children gravitate to the music that their caregivers like. Perhaps they have witnessed some community-based music making, for example, in places of worship or public parks; perhaps they have not. Children are constantly exposed to music on television and video and may assume that those who perform music are glamorous and not ordinary people like themselves. We recommend you include in your intake process a few questions about the child's musical preferences and history of music playing or instruction, if any.

Music in clinical practice is both an interpersonal and an intrapersonal process, and for psychotherapists not familiar with engaging in music pursuits, there is an element of risk taking involved. As mentioned earlier, having confidence in your ability to bring music into the therapy room is critical to success: your client will immediately sense your level of comfort. In both music and psychotherapy, pacing and timing are of utmost importance. The child's needs and impulses lead the way, while their inner resources and ego strength shape the intensity, depth, and form of strategies employed (Crenshaw, 2006). Begin simply and build in complexity or depth as you and your client move into making music. It is more important to quickly establish a safe therapeutic environment than to create a detailed or intricate plan.

This chapter provides information to help therapists and other professionals incorporate musical experiences and activities into a session so that a client feels empowered and in touch with his emotions in a safe and contained manner. It covers how music can be integrated with other therapeutic approaches and describes key skills such as how to listen attentively, how to talk about music, and what to do when powerful emotions or behaviors are evoked through musical play. It ends with a discussion of key issues in treatment, specifically emotion regulation and resistance, where music can play a unique role in working toward healthier ways for children to express themselves and control their responses.

USING MUSIC WITH DIFFERENT THERAPEUTIC APPROACHES

Music can be incorporated in all therapeutic approaches, both verbal and nonverbal. When working with children, therapists may use an eclectic approach, perhaps combining different media in the creative arts such as music, art, drama, and dance/movement. What is chosen and how it is incorporated depends on both the inclination and the skill of the therapist and the needs of the child.

Traditional evidence-based approaches to psychotherapy have at their philosophical core a view of children as products of their pathology, dysfunction, and illness (Ruud, 2010), while more contemporary perspectives view the child as a dynamic, integrated system (DeRobertis, 2008). When a psychotherapist seeks to include some form of musical interaction in therapy, it is useful to understand music as a process that can encapsulate and put into sound the identity of a client and bring another layer of stability into the therapy room. Rather than focusing on children's challenges, limitations, or what they *cannot* do, we instead focus on developing children's strengths and build upon what they *can* do. Taking a strength-based approach allows the child's natural affinity for music to surface and flourish.

We find a humanistic approach to therapy can guide the therapist in establishing a warm and inviting setting. Creating an environment that fosters therapeutic interaction, what DeRobertis calls "lived-space" (2008, p. 151), means establishing a sense of safety in the room through active engagement. This provides an "experiential opening or clearing that invites involvement within the concrete world of things and others" (DeRobertis, 2008, p. 151). The expressive therapies are a powerful means of engaging children in this way.

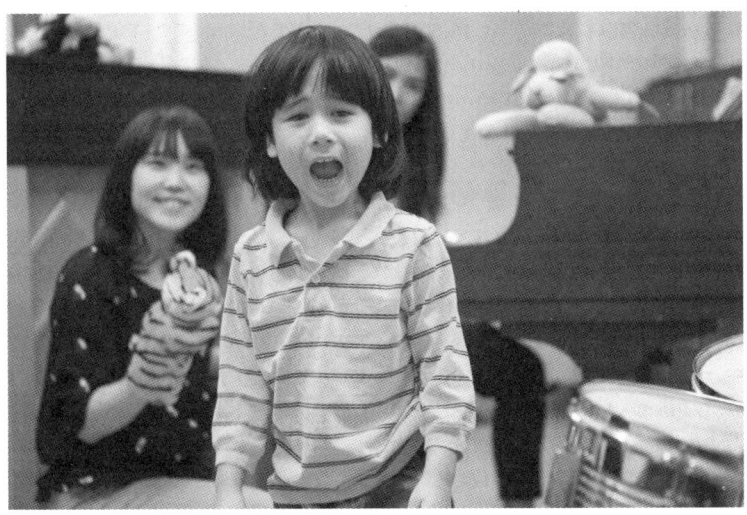

Boy singing with therapists

Music and Play

Therapists who specialize in the use of play may want to consider how to add music (and other creative arts) into their practice. There are many parallels between the use of music and play in therapy, and the two forms of treatment are compatible and complementary. Play is an essential part of developing healthy relationships as well as inner resiliency. It is a physical, creative, explorative process that enhances cognition and ego strength, and boosts the capacity to bond with others. As a therapeutic intervention, play helps children feel heard, understood, and accepted without conditions placed on them (Bratton & Swan, 2017). Playfulness is also an important quality to have when working with children. Being playful encourages a child to become engaged and "conveys a light optimism and confidence in the dialogue and general nonverbal interactions" (Hughes, 2014, p. 109). It invites emotional closeness, imparts a sense of acceptance, and has the capacity to profoundly change children. Trevarthan and Panksepp (2017) state that play changes our genetic profile by stimulating the entire neocortex. A child engaged in healthy, playful interactions that are "punctuated by laughter" experiences pleasure (Trevarthan & Panksepp, 2017, p. 34). Conversely, suppressing or inhibiting the instinct to play can lead to disruptive behaviors.

Making music is in and of itself a form of play: it increases self-confidence, offers a means to explore emotions safely, and builds or rebuilds social connections through cooperation and being with another in the present moment. We play music, either alone or as part of a group. To play authentically requires a child or adult to reach deep into himself and to link personal emotional energy to the melody, rhythm, and harmony of the composition or improvisation. The contour of a melody reflects an emotional process that is uniquely human (Storr, 1991) and "we start to look and feel better when we listen to melodies" (Porges, 2010, p. 8). There is no such thing as a static melody—melody is in constant motion. It is moving either in tonal lines or rhythm, just as life constantly moves and swirls around us. The involvement of motoric, emotional, and creative processes when making music enhances its symbolic power to reflect the child's self. Bringing music into the therapeutic relationship allows the child yet another means by which to symbolically act and interact in a way that is audible and situated in the present moment.

Through play and through music, therapists can provide children with opportunities to express their emotions and use creative problem solving to address real-life concerns in a secure and nurturing environment. Both play and music are universal. Play is the "language" of children: through play, they explore different attitudes and behaviors and try to make sense of their world (Kottman, 2001). Music is generally considered a universal phenomenon in the sense that all people share a capacity to engage in musical expression. Both music and play are projective forms of expression: children project their feelings into their play and into their music. Children communicate symbolically through both their music and their play, imbuing them with meaning (Birnbaum, 2013). They use their play and their music as metaphors to represent themselves and their thoughts, fantasies, feelings, and life circumstances.

Music and Movement/Dance

Movement and dance are forms of expression natural to children, and as adult clinicians we sometimes have to work to reconnect with this spirit. Children literally jump for joy, while adults refer to this as a metaphor for being happy. Human beings have deep connections to dance and movement as primal forms of not just joy and connection, but also of ways to express grief, enact rituals, and build community (Perry, 2008). Music and dance are intertwined, for rhythm enlivens both. When we listen to music, we instinctively move our bodies, whether it be swaying to a waltz or tapping a foot to a catchy beat. When bringing music into the treatment room, be prepared for the child to move—he may naturally want to move his body to the music or even move around the room. This is not a form of restlessness but rather a creative and visceral response to rhythm, tone, and harmony. Moving might help the child expend excess energy and likely will not interfere with the listening or playing experience.

Both music and dance can be solitary, interpersonal, or community pursuits. Like music therapy, dance/movement therapy (DMT) is a creative, clinical modality that reaches deep into the human experience in order to bring succor, healing, and connection. In DMT, artistic expression merges with psychotherapeutic principles to create greater awareness of ourselves as beings who, even as young children, hold memories of joy, sadness, trauma, and love in our bodies (Zubala & Karkou, 2015). DMT interventions often focus on clients who have trouble using words to express themselves and need an emotional outlet. Music and dance overlap in many ways, and when integrated, a rich experience is created for the child, full of creative possibility. Bringing scarves into the session, for example, and dancing with your client allows you to share a connection that needs no words. In this case you could follow how the child moves without exactly imitating it, capturing the quality of his responses to the music, or you could create your own dance that contrasts and complements how the child moves.

Using props such as stretch bands and play parachutes may inspire children to use their bodies in new ways. Games involving listening to music and stopping ('freezing') or striking creative poses when the music stops help children increase their body awareness and regulate their impulses. The 'freeze' game can be enacted with a hand drum or conga drum: when the therapist beats the drum the child moves (typically this is predetermined, often walking or dancing). When the drum beat stops unexpectedly, the child freezes his position until the drum sounds again. Once the rules of the game are clear, roles of who plays the drum and who freezes can be switched back and forth between therapist and client.

THERAPEUTIC SKILLS

Many techniques in child psychotherapy have analogous music techniques. A therapist might paraphrase what a client has said to assure him that she was listening and hearing his message; this is known as *restating content* (Kottman, 2001). Similarly, in music, a therapist can take up or repeat a child's melodic or rhythmic idea to communicate the same thing; this is known as *mirroring* (Isenberg, 2015). When making clinical decisions, therapists using music, play, or other media often rely on intuition as well as careful observation of the child's response to the music or their statements (Birnbaum, 2013). Child psychotherapists use the technique of *reflecting feelings*, making guesses or statements about what they imagine their clients are feeling to help their clients become more aware of their feelings (Kottman, 2001). The musical equivalent of this, or musical reflection, occurs when we observe a child's affect and body language, and use music that reflects the child's mood (Birnbaum, 2013). If a child seems thoughtful or withdrawn, for example, the therapist might choose music with an introspective mood to match the child's feeling. When choosing music, the purpose is not to cheer the child up, but rather to support and enhance the client's feeling.

LISTENING AND BEING FULLY PRESENT

Listening is a crucial part of any therapist's training and clinical approach. However, working with children and music requires deep listening, that is, listening not just to what the child says or plays, but *how* he says or plays it. In Chapter 2, we described how careful observation during musical improvisation can reveal vital information about the child client. The therapist should also carefully observe body language and see how this matches the child's words, for children are often unable to put into words what they are feeling. For example, one child spoke softly in school, never raising her voice above a whisper. When a school psychologist offered her two stuffed animals, however, she took them and pushed them into the floor with force. Her subdued tone of voice suggested anxiety or fear, yet her actions spoke of anger. Movements, gestures, and tone of voice imbue words with meaning. When layers of trauma, distrust, or disability are added into the mix, verbalizing feelings becomes impossible for many children. Children instinctively know whom they can trust, and meeting with someone who has the ability to listen without judgment is something they sense and take comfort in.

Being present and fully active is critical to successfully bringing music into the room. Be ready to abandon something if it does not feel right, but also be aware of any tendency to stop an exercise because you think it does not 'sound good.' Giving a client time to work with the instruments and the activity may mean you at times must expect harsh, loud, or unfamiliar sounds; this type of experimentation is a wonderful way for a child to discover how to make something sound pleasing or satisfying to him. All children need to develop feelings of mastery and to have a means of self-expression, and music experiences are uniquely able to provide these.

Sometimes what we need to do most of all is to simply be present and act as a witness to the child's spontaneous musical expression. He may need to feel in control of the situation, and may not want the therapist to join in. The pace must be determined by the child in order not to overwhelm him or risk retraumatizing him. By providing a safe physical and emotional space, we communicate that we are there to listen to and accept the child's feelings. We can hold the rawest and most tender expressions of feeling, without judgment. When children feel heard, they feel valued; feelings of shame or unworthiness can be transformed into self-esteem and pride. If a therapist's own feelings of insecurity or unease creep into a musical exchange, the child will sense it and quickly retreat. Staying present and attuned to internal shifts helps sustain the safety of the experience.

Letting Go of Biases and Personal Preferences

Accepting our clients for who they are can also mean accepting the music they listen to. This may require us to let go of our own biases and preferences. We may not like a certain type of music, be it rap or classical, country or heavy metal, but if we communicate this dislike, the client may feel that you have rejected a vital part of him. There is a balance between being authentic, meaning not pretending to like something that we do not, and striving to be open and accepting. Communicating respect for a client's musical tastes is crucial to building a trusting relationship.

Adolescents especially may be mistrustful or challenge the authority of adults, and this can be reflected in their preferred music choices. I (J. C. B.) worked with a teenage girl who was exploring her love of singing. As is typical of many teenagers, she was immersed in current music, including rap. She wanted to share with me her mastery of some popular rap songs, but the lyrics were filled with obscenities and vulgar words. She told me that her mother did not allow her to sing the songs at home, and looked at me, waiting to see if I would allow her to sing them in a therapy session. Personally, I do not care for most rap music, particularly songs with misogynistic or violent lyrics. Nevertheless, I told her that there was no censorship in the therapy room and that she was free to sing whatever she chose. My usual stance in individual therapy is to accept all that the client offers as potential material to work on, provided there are no safety issues. She smiled and proceeded to sing a few rap songs—we laughed together at the off-color lyrics. Sharing a musical experience that was otherwise "taboo" helped us to feel closer. She understood that I was not there to judge her or her musical preferences, but rather to support her efforts to express herself as a singer.

It is important to note that my response might have been different had this occurred in a group situation. I would have needed to evaluate the motivation of the client for choosing the song, and the impact that the words might have on other group members. Was the singer being provocative, trying to shock others, and if so, why? Might the lyrics cause offense or be upsetting to other group members? Would this present a good opportunity to open a meaningful discussion, for example, on societal perceptions and expectations of men and women? Or did other group members need protection from what might be interpreted as a verbal attack? In a group setting it is essential to establish ground rules for behavior, spelling out what is acceptable and what is not, inclusive of music lyrics. Consequences for breaching these ground rules must also be clear. Another consideration is the culture of the treatment setting. For example, if the group takes place in a hospital, the therapist must be aware of and comply with the hospital's rules, boundaries, and expectations.

By the time a child is receiving therapy, he has had countless experiences with music at home, in school, and in the larger world. He may have negative associations with music because of a strict or insensitive music teacher, who perhaps berated him for playing or singing wrong notes. We have heard of choral teachers telling some children to stand in the back and not sing, as they did not meet the teachers' standards. In situations where the arts are viewed as a "frill," it may be acceptable to punish a child by excluding him from musical experiences or performances. Children who have difficulty taking direction or working as part of an ensemble may be banned from participating in musical experiences in school. All of these common scenarios communicate failure to the child and can cause him to feel that any musical expression is outside his reach. By bringing music into the therapy room in a creative and thoughtful way, we provide positive experiences for children that may change their feelings about music and about themselves.

HOW TO TALK ABOUT MUSIC

Knowing what to say about music and how to frame its place in therapy with children is as important as knowing how to incorporate musical elements into clinical practice. Music evokes powerful responses in clients and saying too much or too little can decrease the therapeutic potential present in the moments following a musical interaction or shared listening experience. Our general guideline is to err on the side of caution and say *less* than you might think you need to. Allowing the child to have an unmediated response to the music, whether it is emotional, a charged memory, or simply a lessening of feeling, sends a message of trust. Music has the power to prompt the desire to interact without the need for verbal reinforcement. That said, knowing how to contextualize, sustain, and support a child's musical expression using words may increase how deeply the child will feel the effects.

Using language geared to a child's developmental and cognitive level is essential. Language that is clear and consistent will increase a child's feeling of security. Be aware of using words or phrases that can sound threatening. Saying "Hit the drum" might lead a child to think hitting is okay. You could use the words *tap* or *strike* instead. Using correct names for instruments is beneficial to fostering respect and increasing self-efficacy. For example, using the term "mallet" instead of "beater" for the sticks used to play a drum gives a sense of formality and mastery. Saying "djembe" instead of tall drum gives the drum an identity.

We also recommend that you do not mention your own feelings about the child's music in more than a minimally supportive manner.

Repeated statements such as "I like the way you did that" might cause a child to feel that he is expected to please you. The goal is for music making to be intrinsically rewarding, such that the child should not become dependent on our praise for validation. It is instinctive to respond to a client's music making by saying "Good!," "Nice job," or some similar words of praise. Saying "That was good" or "That sounded great" is a bland response that does not highlight the child's engagement. The word *interesting* falls into this category as well and is one we try to avoid. Using these kinds of words implies that we are judging the child's music, and, by extension, the child himself. Children in psychotherapy may have been told repeatedly, whether verbally or through nuanced behavior, that they are somehow defective. It is the therapist's job to consistently and kindly disavow this type of internalized assumption. Once a relationship has been established, there are times when it would be acceptable—and therapeutic—to share an authentic feeling with a child, but this must be done with care. It is always helpful to take a moment to think about how your message might be received.

VIGNETTE

I (L. E. B.) worked with Len, a 3-year-old boy with significant developmental and cognitive issues. His mother said he was constantly frustrated because of his inability to make himself understood. Len was a friendly child who enthusiastically engaged in music making. One day, after finishing a short improvisation, Len shouted out "GOOD,!" then turned to me, beaming. He shouted this again after singing a different song, and it dawned on me that he had taken on my response to him—each time we finished playing I had been saying "Good!" loudly and energetically. On the one hand, I felt I had set Len up for feeling badly if he did not think the music sounded good. On the other hand, I realized that Len was affirming his innate goodness over and over. When his mother saw him on videotape proudly exclaiming "GOOD!," she became emotional and told me that it was wonderful to see him saying something positive about himself, for he had already been told so many times in his young life that he was not doing things well, or that he was somehow off-track. For Len, this internalization of "GOOD!" had a therapeutic effect, yet I realized that my tendency to say this word in response to any music a client made could dilute its meaning. That experience marked a turning point: I knew from then on, I needed to be truthful yet supportive in my comments and avoid using words that were charged with expectation or laden with emotion. Saying "good" implied that bad music was possible. Fortunately, I learned this lesson with a child who needed to completely own his power and ability to make music that sounded good to him.

Here are some examples of objective, specific, and useful comments to consider after a client plays or sings:

- "This is the first time we ended our playing at the same time." [Focus on beginning or ending.]
- "The beginning of the piece was _____, while the ending sounded _____." [Focus on beginning or ending.]
- "That one part where you sang (fill in a lyric or a piece of the melody) _____ was different from the rest of the song." [Here you could suggest that the child repeat the music, sing or play it back to them, or ask why he thinks it was different.]
- "I thought your playing sounded stronger this session than last session." [Link playing to a previous way of playing.]
- "When you first started playing you weren't looking at the drum, but as you kept playing you started to look at where the mallet struck the drum." [Reflect on what the client did.]
- "Your voice while singing was clear and powerful." [Make a non-judgmental comment that highlights positive aspects of singing.]
- "When you were singing the second verse your voice cracked a little, and it really matched what the words were saying." [Link vocal quality to the lyrics.]
- "I noticed how you sang that phrase a little softer than the other phrases." [Reflect changes in vocal intensity.]
- "You switched playing instruments in the middle of our playing, and I was wondering what you were thinking when you did that." [Ask why the client made a change.]
- "Do you think we could try something different next time?" [Solicit ideas for future play.]

This leads us to the question of what words to use to describe the music. There are many descriptive words possible, yet there are some that frequently come up in our own practice that capture how music sounds without layering any kind of judgment onto it. We cannot overemphasize the importance of being genuine and honest when reflecting on a client's choice of music or musical play. Clients, especially children, know when we are placating them. The key here is to focus on what was played, how it was played, or on specific elements of the music.

There are different approaches you can use in talking about the music. Taking the fill-in option discussed above of "The beginning of the piece was _____," here are some options when working with older children: energizing/steady; sad/upbeat; soft/harsh; chaotic/peaceful; uplifting/somber; intense/quiet; and exciting/smooth. These words focus on qualities of the music that you might think of or experience when listening. Tapping into your own candid reactions is a good place to start. If you are working with a young child, using simpler words can capture the essence of the music, such as loud/big, slow/sad, or fast/happy.

When referring to music in emotional terms, it is important to simply identify how it felt or sounded without implying it is how the client feels. The phrase "It sounded _____" is one that has served us well. You can interject many different terms here: happy, sad, angry, joyful, safe, tentative, strong, meek, vulnerable, open, closed-down, ambiguous, chaotic, intense, or inviting, to name a few. Since feelings about music are so subjective, you might pick up on an emotion that the client does *not* share. That is absolutely fine—if your client tells you that he thought or felt something different, it is best to simply acknowledge this difference. For example, if you said, "It sounded sad" and your client says, "I thought it sounded happy," you might reply, "It sounded sad to me, but you heard the music differently and thought it sounded happy. Did it make you feel happy?," or "What was it about the music that sounded happy?" There are many possible explanations for this kind of discrepancy: you might be projecting your own feelings onto the music, the client may be consciously or unconsciously avoiding his own uncomfortable feelings, or it may simply be a matter of individual differences and preferences. After all, there is no "right way" to hear or describe music. The information gleaned from these observations, however, can inform the therapeutic process. Having a different perspective of the music and voicing this can be a surprise to the child and, if pragmatically and thoughtfully phrased, can increase his ability to tolerate others' responses.

Another strategy is to refer to the musical elements we reviewed in Chapter 1. Just as when we talk about a picture using words that describe color, line, shape, or composition (Malchiodi, 1998), we use language that describes the components of music. You might focus on the melody and say it was flowing, full of leaps, predictable, edgy, lyrical, sharp, or that it somehow suited the words. This opens the door to asking the client what he thought about the melody and having a conversation about this unique element of the piece. When talking about the rhythm of a piece of music, you can say it was steady or unpredictable, driving or soothing, jumpy or smooth. Since rhythm is felt in the body, observe any spontaneous movement your client may do—rocking or swaying, toe tapping—and discuss how the music makes him feel like moving. In addition, mirroring or responding to the movement with a similar movement can serve to support, reflect back, and validate the child's response to the music.

When speaking about timbre, or the quality of the sound, you can consider whether the music sounded gentle or strong, rounded or thin, warm or harsh, mellow or shrill, dark or bright, heavy or light. Sometimes timbre evokes images: organ music might evoke an image of ice skating or a wedding; brass instruments might bring up an image of a parade. With respect to dynamics, or volume, we can talk about more than just the loudness or softness of the music. What is the intensity and expressive quality? Does it start softly and build up to a climax, or does the music gently fade away? Do dynamics change gradually, or are they sudden and take you by surprise? Are there strong accented notes that are exciting and seem to propel the music forward? You might comment, "I heard you changing from loud to soft playing during the song." You can also discuss the overall feel of a piece of music: was it soothing or stimulating, beautiful or ugly?

When a piece finishes, reflecting on the way it affected you encourages the client to share his reaction. Being authentic in our responses may mean we need to reveal parts of who we are as people, not just as the child's therapist. When a song or instrumental piece is beautiful, it is evident, it is felt. Acknowledging this can be deeply satisfying for a child, for it is a human response to an aesthetically moving moment. The acknowledgment may come through verbal expression, or it might simply be sitting in silence together for a few moments. This type of silence is charged with relational importance, for this bonding moment between client and therapist is visceral and emotional at the same time. It is also a way to acknowledge that sometimes words cannot say what we feel.

VIGNETTE

Troy, a school counselor, had been seeing Cara, a 13-year-old who was struggling with a recent diagnosis of dyslexia, for 2 months. Cara was ambivalent about therapy: on the one hand, she was eager to learn why school was so hard for her; on the other hand, she was angry about being singled out for counseling and for needing extra attention.

One day, Troy was sitting at his desk, writing up notes on his computer and listening to Arvo Pärt, an Estonian composer. The piece

"Spiegel im Spiegel" was playing when Cara appeared at his door, looking upset and saying, "I know it's not our time to meet, but can we talk?" He gestured to her to come in and sit down. She asked, "What is that music? It sounds like it's on a mountaintop." Troy shared the name with her and turned the sound up a few levels so it could be heard more clearly yet not be overwhelming. They lapsed into silence and listened to the remaining 4 minutes of the piece. During this time Cara's facial expression softened and her breathing became more even. When the piece finished, she commented, "That was cool." Troy responded, "This music helps me feel calmer. Do you feel calmer?" Cara replied, "Yeah, a little bit. Maybe I need that piece on my playlist." Troy wanted to encourage her to say more, so he elaborated, "I liked how peaceful it sounded. What did you think of it?" Cara said, "Yeah, it was peaceful, wasn't it? It just made me stop thinking for a while. I liked it." The composition of the piece has simplicity at its core, in which the violin holds long tones over the steady harmony of the piano, creating a soothing effect. Troy saw the shift in Cara's mood, and realized that just listening to the music helped her feel more grounded. Her demeanor in talking with him about an upsetting incident did not have the angry charge she initially had when entering the room. Her emotional state had changed as a result of listening to the music.

In subsequent sessions their interactions were more direct, and Troy felt the therapeutic relationship strengthening. Cara made eye contact more frequently, shared some details about her home life without seeming as nervous as before, and often brought up the topic of music with Troy. The experience of listening to a piece together was not replicated, but its after-effects had a positive impact on their relationship.

MUSIC AS AN AFFIRMATION OF THE CHILD

Children in treatment often feel that they have continually made mistakes in their lives and that they are destined to keep messing up. One of the benefits of bringing music into therapy is that it is a place where it is okay to make mistakes; if the music does not sound "good" right away, with work it will get better. Often the work it takes to make music sound better is minimal—simply holding a mallet differently to play an instrument, or standing up instead of sitting to sing, can make an immediate and positive impact on the sound being produced. Reinforcing this understanding with clients can happen naturally in music; with focused attention, music sounds increasingly satisfying. Or the focus might shift from trying to make music that sounds "good" to making music that embodies a different quality: strength, discord, humor, fear, or joy. A small shift such as moving to a song that is in a minor key to create a sad sound, or speeding up the music to create a happy sound, can make a difference.

What could be interpreted as a mistake in music very often enhances the overall sound: dissonance (meaning a combination of tones that sounds unharmonious or clashing), in small doses, can bring vitality and healthy tension to a piece. If you are listening to music with a young client, you can talk about dissonant parts of the music in this way: "What did that music make you think of?" Or "How did this music feel to you?" Or even "Did you think of a certain place or a person while listening?" With an adolescent client you may be able to use more sophisticated language: "What made this part of the music sound strong?"; "Does the discord or conflict show a different kind of feeling?" or, more directly, "I wonder if the tension in the music reminds you of any conflicts in your own life?" These questions and how the child or teen responds emotionally become mirrors for how a child feels about himself.

MUSIC AND EMOTION REGULATION

Emotion regulation is the ability of a person to effectively modulate his feelings and control when and how he experiences them, while emotion dysregulation is "the lack of temper control, affective lability, and emotional overreaction" (Cavanagh, Quinn, Duncan, Graham, & Balbuena, 2017, p. 381). With its intrinsic ability to organize thoughts and actions through rhythm and melody, music gives the child a natural form to consolidate his impulses so he can make satisfying sounds and makes it possible for the child to learn how to self-soothe and regulate (Robarts, 2014). The process of playing or even just listening to music requires a child or teenager to regulate his emotions to engage successfully. As structured sound, music affords a way for the child to vent, process, and understand his own emotions. When playing with a therapist, the child is doing these things while also interacting with another person: the music is a unitive force that brings them together (Kossak, 2009).

In the neurosequential model of therapeutics, Gaskill and Perry (2014) emphasize the importance of repetitive and rewarding experiences in altering the neural systems involved in the stress response.

They note how music, dance, walking, and similar rhythmic and patterned activities are inherently soothing and can be seen as a "primal language" that changes the primary regulatory networks in the lower brain (Gaskill & Perry, 2014, p. 187). A clinical approach based on developmentally appropriate activities helps children regulate their emotions and enhances their relational and cognitive abilities (Perry, 2008). Using music in an environment of safety, enjoyment, and attunement is a powerful, nonverbal means of accessing the child's regulatory networks and provides the groundwork for the healing process.

Children are often referred to therapy or counseling because of problematic or disruptive behaviors, yet these behaviors serve a function: they are often a child's only defense and a means of protecting himself against painful emotions and a world he does not understand. When a child is in a state of emotional distress, he becomes either hyperaroused or dissociated from his surroundings (Schore, 2009; Siegel, 2006). When in a safe environment, it becomes possible for music's naturally analgesic effects to counter this physiological response. Music can help the child begin to learn to regulate his emotional states in a natural, noninvasive manner (Kossak, 2009). Further, the therapist can shift the musical elements to fit the needs of the child. As an example, Michelyn, a 13-year-old girl with developmental delays, would become overstimulated and would throw herself on the ground and scream, "I want to go home!" over and over. When I (L. E. B.) started working with her in an afterschool program, I was startled by the intensity and sustained nature of her outburst. I knew her favorite song was "The Wheels on the Bus," so I went over to her, leaned down, and softly sang the song. She immediately sat up, started singing with me but in a fast way, and got up so that we were walking and singing together. After we had sung the song many times, I deliberately slowed the tempo down and Michelyn followed suit. She slowed her singing to a more natural pace and we matched our footsteps to the rhythm. She calmed down and we returned to the group. Over the course of several weeks we continued to work on singing when she became distressed as well as slowing her singing down. Staff remarked she became calmer in other situations during the program as well.

A brief example of work on an inpatient child psychiatric unit illustrates the power of music to shape an environment in order to contain, stimulate, or calm children with significant emotional difficulties. Clinicians on the unit requested our help on how to incorporate music into the daily routine of the children without it being overwhelming or overstimulating. After careful observation and discussion, we decided to focus on transitions, especially to and from lunch. The children were prone to excitability in coming to the lunchroom as they had been in "quiet time" in their own rooms for an hour preceding the meal. After lunch, the children went to recreation and tended to run down the hallway to get there. After observing these periods of transition, it was clear that the children had pent-up energy and no immediate, constructive way of managing it. We wanted to acknowledge their feelings of excitement without elevating the level of activity. We decided to focus on theme songs taken from movies we knew the children especially liked, such as *Superman* and *Star Wars*. The music that John Williams composed for these movies is powerful in its effect and is quickly recognized. There are also no words in these pieces, something we felt was important. We wanted the children to feel the power, majesty, and beauty of the music, yet did not want to engage their desire to sing along as this can be distressing to certain sound-sensitive children. The staff members decided to play the *Star Wars* theme while going to lunch, and *Superman* when heading to recreation time. The music was piped over the loudspeaker at a moderate volume, and it quickly became the signal for these transitions. Instead of having to talk loudly, clap hands, or otherwise get the children's attention, simply playing the music immediately got their attention and they either came out of the rooms to wait for a line to be formed or took their trays to the bussing area and lined up to go to recreation time. Staff members noted that, while it was not always effective, the music helped to modulate these otherwise chaotic and disruptive times of day and had become highlights of the children's experience on the unit. It lightened the mood while simultaneously orienting everyone to the transition at hand.

USING MUSIC TO ADDRESS RESISTANCE IN THERAPY

As all therapists know, children do not always cooperate with goals and expectations in the therapy setting. A child who resists participating in a session presents unique challenges for the therapist (Baron, 2014). Malchiodi and Crenshaw (2017) point out that, historically speaking, referring to a child as being resistant is a form of blaming the child for not participating. This is counterproductive to the goals of treatment. Their work advances the idea that children avoid therapeutic interventions not out of any conscious intention, but rather because there are neurobehavioral, cognitive, and/or emotional issues that prevent them from engaging (2017). Understanding the many underlying factors, whether neurobehavioral, cognitive, cultural, familial, or developmental, helps therapists approach the work with a more child-centered and positive approach. Creative therapies that are essentially nondirective and nonverbal in nature can be a powerful way of dealing with resistance: "When children cannot tell their story in words, even those as young as three can express their inner worlds through play, art, sand tray creations, or other creative arts depictions" (Malchiodi & Crenshaw, 2017, p. 8).

Music therapists Nordoff and Robbins understood resistance (they use the term "resistiveness") as a lens through which to assess a child's ability to engage in therapy. Their early work in the 1960s was ahead of its time in that they viewed resistance in a positive light without judging the child's response. Nordoff and Robbins (2007) formulated a scale for assessing resistance based on the idea that the resistive responses of the child are often a corollary to participation. Just as there are levels of participation that progress through recognizable stages, there are levels of resistiveness with distinct qualities ranging from active rejection to assertive contesting. Resistance can be subtle or overt. For example, the child may cry or tantrum, or run away or hide from the therapist. He may ignore or try to shut out the therapist. These behaviors are indicative of a low level of engagement. Alternately, the child may stop playing with the therapist, or try to prevent the therapist from playing, or try to control his actions. The latter often takes the form of teasing, which is a higher level of interaction than avoidance. The child may use materials in destructive ways, throwing or trying to break things—this demonstrates an active will and response to the environment.

Nordoff and Robbins (2007) raise the question of how to work with resistance, regain cooperation, restore confidence, and facilitate the therapy process. Rather than viewing it as something to conquer, it is more clinically effective to find techniques to work through resistance. By embracing rather than avoiding a child's resistance, the therapist can encourage interaction, deepen a sense of safety and trust, and bypass the impulse to avoid contact.

What might cause this reluctance to participate? There are several possible explanations. What may appear as resistance to therapy is often an expression of the child's inflexibility or discomfort with change of routine, environment, or people in their lives; these types of changes can cause great anxiety. A child may be communicating his frustration or be attempting to self-regulate or protect himself. He may be expressing fear of failure, fear of intimacy, or he may be fearful of music that expresses unconscious thoughts and feelings. A child may be resistant because of a need to control, or anxious about losing control, or simply not able to talk about what he is feeling (VanFleet & Faa-Thompson, 2017). He may be ambivalent about allowing close contact with the therapist due to past traumas or abuse (Crenshaw, 2017). It is important to remember that a child's actions—or inactions—have meaning as well as the potential to become habitual or ingrained behaviors (Nordoff & Robbins, 2007; Steele, 1984).

Many specialists agree that resistance is a natural part of the therapeutic process. According to Austin and Dvorkin (1998), "Resistance is not something to be eliminated but instead offers a way toward understanding the client. It should be seen as a form of communication and respected in the same way" (p. 128). The therapist's job is to meet and work creatively with the child to establish a working alliance and create a safe environment for the child to express himself.

VIGNETTE

For several months Dov, an 8-year-old boy, had been working with Zach, a play therapist. They reached a plateau in the therapy, and Zach decided to try bringing in a keyboard, knowing that his relationship with Dov was one of trust and warmth. Dov had exhibited musical tendencies, yet when Zach began to play the keyboard, Dov resisted. He started to yell at him to stop and pulled his hands from the keys. It quickly became impossible to carry out the activity together. Rather than giving in to Dov's strong efforts to control him, Zach held his ground with quiet and steady determination. When Dov refused to stop grabbing Zach's hands and defiantly yelled out, "No I won't!," Zach countered by playfully repeating, "Yes I will!" in a clear rhythmic pattern, picking out notes to match the rhythm, and matching and even exceeding Dov's intensity. Even though Dov outwardly rejected Zach's attempts to play with him, his musical sensibilities were awakened, and he began to sing more tonally based on the melodies Zach was playing. When he yelled again at Zach to stop, Zach teasingly replied that he could not stop and improvised a song with the lyrics "There's music in my fingers, there's music in my hands, there's music in my feet. . . . there's music everywhere, anywhere. . . . " Dov seemed to see the humor in this and he and Zach engaged in antiphonal (back and forth) singing with the words "everywhere, anywhere." Dov's resistance seemed to melt away as he began to enjoy singing with Zach and sustaining his tones—for example, by singing "muuuuuuusic." The playfulness of the musical interaction with Zach was so engaging that Dov could let go of whatever it was that was causing him to avoid participating, and to join wholeheartedly in the experience. By attuning to Dov's tone of voice and intensity, Zach was able to work with the playful qualities of Dov's resistance and turn them into an interactive game.

SUMMARY

In therapy, the physical and emotional safety of our clients is paramount. In this chapter we have seen examples of how music can be used to help in creating a safe space in which children can flourish. By communicating an attitude of acceptance and being sensitive when talking about music, you can create an atmosphere of safety and emotional security for your clients. Playing or listening to selected music can help a child or adolescent regulate his emotions and experience success. When children resist participating or present challenging behaviors, using music in an interactive, playful way can diffuse the situation and gain the child's cooperation.

RECOMMENDATIONS FOR PRACTICE

For a therapist who is not a musician or is uncertain of how to incorporate music into treatment, we recommend you start simply. Feeling confident and comfortable about what you will be doing is essential to creating a space in which the child will feel safe.

- Borrow or purchase a few small instruments that make different sounds—it is simplest to start with percussion instruments such as a hand drum or tambourine, shaker or bells, and woodblocks. See Chapter 2 for more suggestions and information about instruments.
- Play along with recordings of different kinds of music, exploring different ways of using the instruments and getting the feel of the rhythm.
- If you are self-conscious about singing, listen to recordings of a wide variety of songs and hum along. During your day, create chants about what you are doing—taking a walk, cooking dinner—using whatever

rhythm comes to mind. You can also make up chants about other people and even your pets!
- Consider role playing with a friend or colleague. Take turns playing different kinds of clients—a child who is excitable, angry, depressed, or fearful, for example—and try to reflect and support them using the available instruments and/or your voice. This type of peer collaboration can quickly build your confidence.

When Creating Safe Space

- Have music playing in the waiting room that is geared specifically to the child's musical preferences. You will, however, want to avoid this step unless you are able to identify songs that do not have violent or misogynistic lyrics. Playing themes from recent popular movies can help the client feel at ease.
- When in the treatment room, if the child is verbal, ask him what he thought of the music that had been playing in the waiting room. This can help establish rapport.

When Working on Emotion Regulation

- When working with an emotionally labile child, taking your attention off him and focusing instead on the music or instrument can redirect the child's energy. A child who is worked up emotionally and has a degree of self-awareness may try to pull another person into his state, and when a therapist does not meet the emotional intensity but diverts his attention to a different yet satisfying venture, the child is given a way to de-escalate. He has the opportunity to express his curiosity about what the therapist is doing or playing; sometimes the child will try to stop the therapist from this diversion and take the instrument or ask the therapist to stop. Whatever the therapist does next, the child has shifted into a different state of communication, of his own volition.

When Working with a Child Who Is Resistant

- Avoid argument and direct confrontation. Try taking a gently humorous, coaxing approach in working to overcome resistance and invite participation. Treat resistance playfully as a means of communication. For example, if the child refuses to do something, make a game out of singing *no, no, no, yes, yes, yes*.

- Meeting the child's level of emotional intensity in playing or singing or choosing a piece to listen to that matches this intensity can serve as a release of energy for the child. In the work Zach did with Dov, Zach mirrored Dov's energy back to him but was able, by creating a call-and-response type of musical interaction, to give Dov the means to de-escalate his resistance and move it into a more playful and healthy exchange.
- Add inflection to your speaking voice and exaggerate the melody contained in the phrases and patterns. This brings a sing-song quality to speech that children naturally respond to and often want to engage in. It also shifts the therapist away from unconsciously taking a controlling or punitive tone of voice in trying to manage the child's behavior.
- Put emphasis on the child's reality rather than on your own agenda. Avoid assuming the role of "expert"; we may not have all the answers. If we are fixed in our ideas and expect the child to comply, we are setting the stage for resistance. For example, it is best not to insist that he sing a song, even though you think it might be helpful for him. If we assume a stance of openness there will be less for the child to resist.
- When you encounter resistance, slow the pace of the words, music, or interaction. If a child wants to sing the same song 20 times (like Michelyn), that is okay. It might seem repetitive and tedious to you, but it likely has a very different meaning for the child. A child who perseverates or becomes obsessive requires different interventions. As the therapist, you will interpret the child's behavior and the reasons behind it, based on your observations and your knowledge of the child's history and issues, and make clinical decisions accordingly. Try introducing small changes in volume, tempo, or lyrics, as even small changes can present big challenges for such children. If repeating songs or phrases seems perseverative, redirecting to a different sound or an alternative play therapy approach might be called for. Finding ways to transition in and out of obsessive tendencies is part of treatment for some children.
- Express empathy through reflective listening and accept the child's feelings. Remember that the child is not simply being stubborn; there is a reason for his behavior (Steele, 1984). Pay close attention to his body language, the rhythm of his movements, his sounds and vocal quality, and pick up on what seems most significant.

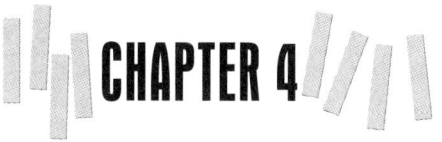

CHAPTER 4

Music in Child Development

> All clients, regardless of areas of need, can experience the potential for transformation at the heart of musical development, either through active music-making or receptive listening.
> —AIGEN (2014, p. 23)

Human beings grow, learn, and develop by playing, whether alone or with others. In Chapter 3 we introduced the idea of play as having multiple interpretations. The idea of play is embedded in its various meanings in the very action of making music: we *play* music. For children who are in some way inhibited in their growth or ability to express themselves, making music stimulates a sense of purposeful, in-the-moment engagement that can help them reach new developmental milestones. Taking part in musical experiences inspires creativity and prompts sensations of joy, perseverance, and happiness. Having fun while playing is essential to healthy development for any child, and music naturally invokes spontaneity and a sense of pleasurable involvement. Music touches all areas of development: physical, emotional, intellectual, spiritual, and social (Harvey, 2017). Each of these areas is vital for healthy development and a positive sense of self.

The development of musical ability is as natural to children as the development of language, for they have many cognitive mechanisms in common (Patel, 2017). Language acquisition and cognitive development are processes often paralleled by a child's ability to attune to sounds and rhythms, distinguish voices and pitches, sing, and play instruments. Current psychological and neurological theories support the notion that children are hardwired to integrate, understand, and grow both linguistically and musically (Hodges & Sebald, 2011). In this chapter we provide a foundation for how clinicians and educators can incorporate music into their work in ways that are appropriate to the child's stage of development and culture. We explore children's typical musical development including how music can enhance cognitive, emotional, and social development. We also discuss theorists' models of how children develop musically, showing what strategies may work best at each stage. The chapter concludes with a section on the importance of cultural considerations in providing meaningful musical interventions.

TYPICAL DEVELOPMENT

Nineteenth-century philosopher Friedrich Nietzsche is credited with saying "Without music, life would be a mistake" (1889/1990). Indeed, music is so much a part of human experience that it is hard to imagine life without it. Infants are naturally musical beings, cooing melodically and babbling in rhythmic patterns. Language develops from this musicality and it serves as a building block to human communication (Trevarthen, 2002). Let us consider again the effect a lullaby has on an infant, for example. With its activating melody, predictable rhythmic movement, and minimal thematic development, the lullaby invites infants to attune quickly and experience it as a communicative event (Loewy et al., 2013; Trevarthen, 2002).

Hearing is the first sense to develop in the womb. In utero, an infant can hear her mother's heartbeat and other sounds of her mother's body. At 24 weeks' gestation, the fetus has a functional cochlea, the hearing mechanism in the ear (Sherrod, Vietze, & Friedman, 1978). By 32 weeks' gestation, she is able to respond differentially to auditory stimuli varying in intensity and frequency. Many parents intuitively understand the beneficial effects music can have on their baby's development and place headphones on the mother's belly, so that the baby can hear the music and feel the vibrations. We encourage this practice, for research is showing the many positive developmental impacts music has on neonates as well as mothers (González et al., 2017).

At birth, infants respond to the sounds they hear, especially human speech sounds, and are even more responsive to singing (Tsang, Falk, & Hessel, 2017). Condon and Sander (1974) found that infants synchronize their movements to adult speech in a kind of dance of communication. This innate ability of infants and caregivers to attune to one another is further discussed in Chapter 5. Suffice it to say that infants are wired to perceive and attend to the elements of both language and music.

Research shows that newborns as young as 2 days old respond to music (Sherrod et al., 1978). Studies in which babies were provided with music while engaged in nonnutritive sucking showed that they sucked for a longer period of time when the music continued and for a shorter time when the music stopped. The music served as an auditory reinforcement, and results confirmed that the infants heard the music and preferred it (Sherrod et al., 1978).

A newborn baby not only can hear but can distinguish one pitch from another. In one study (Smart & Smart, 1978), a musical note was played while an infant was sucking. The baby stopped sucking to listen, but after hearing the note repeated several times, he habituated and resumed sucking. Yet when a *new* note was played, the baby again stopped sucking, indicating that he recognized that the second note was different from the first: he stopped sucking to attend to the new sound. Other studies have focused on changes in heart rate to indicate discrimination between sounds. Babies react differently to low-pitched sounds, which tend to soothe crying babies and activate alert, calm infants, and high-pitched sounds, which can promote distress. Newborns also react differently to varying levels of volume (Calikusu Incekar & Balci, 2017; Smart & Smart, 1978).

The Benefits of Music

Nobel Prize-winning physicist Albert Einstein credited music with inspiring his most famous discovery: "The theory of relativity occurred to me by intuition, and music is the driving force behind this intuition. My parents had me study the violin from the time I was six. My new discovery is the result of musical perception" (quoted in Suzuki, 1969, p. 90). Interest in understanding the benefits of music has increased over the years and researchers are examining the effects of music education and training on various aspects of development. Mounting evidence supports music's positive effects on early development and the acquisition of specific cognitive skills in the areas of general academic achievement, IQ, reading, mathematics, visual–spatial skills, attention, and memory (Patel, 2017; Winner, Goldstein, & Vincent-Lancrin, 2013). Music can be effective in enhancing children's attentiveness. Taylor (2010) purports, "Musical perception and participation stimulate the brain to organize incoming stimuli and to plan and execute corresponding behavior, thereby enhancing perceptual ability, cognitive processing, and interactive response capability" (p. 103). As children become more focused and organized, they are more receptive to learning and remembering information (Standley, 2002).

Schellenberg (2005) is one of many researchers investigating the relationship between musical and nonmusical abilities. While he found that music listening led to short-term improvement on several cognitive tests, music lessons were associated with relatively long-lasting improvement in children's cognitive abilities that could not be attributed to parents' education and income level. Moreno et al. (2011) studied the short-term effects of music education on verbal intelligence and executive function, and concluded, "Our data have confirmed a rapid transfer of cognitive benefits in young children after only 20 days of music training. The strength of this effect in almost all of the children was remarkable" (quoted in Royal Conservatory of Music, 2014, p. 3). Ninety percent of the children in this study, ages 4 to 6, showed this improvement. Other studies also support the notion that children who take music lessons in addition to their academic curriculum, at least in Western society, have higher IQs than those who do not (Winner et al., 2013). Large-scale studies of school success have found a strong correlation between learning to play a musical instrument and academic achievement (Young, Cordes, & Winner, 2013). The authors note that participation in other arts and sports activities did not yield this positive result.

Music training has been shown to enhance preschool children's spatial–temporal reasoning (Hallam, 2016; Rauscher et al., 1997). Spatial–temporal reasoning involves manipulating mental images and is used in mathematics and science. Rauscher et al. (1997) suggest that "music training produces long-term modifications in underlying neural circuitry in regions not primarily concerned with music" (p. 2). Researchers have uncovered similar positive connections in older children between learning to play music and spatial reasoning, and listening to music and spatial–temporal reasoning (Hetland & Winner, 2004).

Recent research demonstrates a strong link between music and language. Both music and speech are auditory activities that share the same acoustic parameters and involve complex and meaningful sound sequences. In addition, they share the goal of communicating with another human being (Moreno, 2009). Lorenzo, Herrera, Hernandez-Candelas, and Badea (2014) conducted a longitudinal study of the effect of formal musical training on language development in 3- to 4-year-old children and found that music significantly enhances early childhood language development. In another study, Thompson, Schellenberg, and Husain (2004) found that training in music enhances sensitivity to emotions conveyed by speech prosody. Prosody refers to the sound of speech, such as intonation, rhythm, and stress patterns, and how these contribute to meaning. Music education develops listening skills that appear to strengthen the auditory perception of speech sounds and thus stimulate reading skills (Carpentier, Moreno, & McIntosh, 2016; Chen-Haftek & Mang, 2018). Researchers are finding a causal relationship between musical training and word decoding skills (Winner et al., 2013).

In other areas, investigators are studying the influence of music on creativity and interpersonal relationships in children. For example, Passanisi, Di Nuovo, Urgese, and Pirrone (2015) found that 9-year-olds who participated in group musical activities improved in these two areas. The authors suggest that the positive impact of acquiring musical skills, particularly in a group context, has far-reaching implications for student learning, affecting social skills, emotional sensitivity, and creativity. Studies focusing on the social benefits of early musical experiences, including parent–child communication and children's peer relationships, have generally found positive results (Hallam, 2016; Lonie, 2010).

There is danger when focusing on transfer effects—how music making impacts nonmusical abilities—of losing sight of one crucial idea: "The development of musicality as an outcome in itself is a key aspect of infant and early childhood development" (Lonie, 2010, p. 6). Musicality is valuable in and of itself, and the study of emerging communicative musicality needs further attention (Trevarthen, 2002). Research focus needs to be balanced between transfer effects and children's right to musicality and creative expression (Lonie, 2010).

NEUROSCIENCE AND MUSIC

The human brain is one of the most complex creations on our planet. With advancements in brain imaging techniques, scientists are now able to more precisely examine brain structures and anatomical changes (Moreno, 2009). The idea that we are split into left-brain or right-brain personalities, however, is a myth: we may have hemispheric dominance in how we process and assimilate information, yet there are very few, if any, human activities that do not cross over the corpus callosum (Nielson, Zielinski, Ferguson, Lainhart, & Anderson, 2013). The brain is an organ designed to engage fully in music. Much research has been conducted to identify the many areas of the brain involved in music processing: there are certain areas responsible for specific functions (Koelsch, 2012).

Levitin (2007) writes, "Musical activity involves nearly every region of the brain that we know about, and nearly every neural subsystem" (pp. 85–86). Research on the connection between music, neurological functioning, and learning supports behavioral outcomes such as those described in the preceding section.

It is well established that humans use shared brain areas in processing music and language (Patel, 2008; Winner et al., 2013). Moreno, a neuroscientist studying how music impacts the brains of children, states, "Musical training impacts a set of processes in the brain that are related to a whole host of other activities, from intelligence to reading to the ability to focus and do well in school. . . . Music is an incredibly powerful tool, we're learning" (in Royal Conservatory of Music, 2014, p. 4). Music works across cortical areas to strengthen verbal and memory skills (Cheung, Chan, Liu, Law, & Wong, 2017) and stimulates a desire to move (Levitin, Grahn, & London, 2018). Learning how to read and play music has an effect on the anatomical and functional organization of the brain and enhances auditory perception of speech as well as pitch discrimination in music. Moreno et al. (2009) found that after a 24-week period of music instruction, children's auditory discrimination and ability to read inconsistent words improved. They measured electrophysiological effects using event-related potentials (ERPs); ERPs measure electrical activity in the brain in response to complex cognitive tasks. The greater ERP response in the children supports the behavioral findings. Trainor, Shahin, and Roberts (2003) looked at brain activity in 4- to 5-year-old children before and after a year's violin instruction in the Suzuki method. Those who had received the training had a significantly more developed auditory cortex compared to children who had not received the training, which means they were able to discriminate between a greater number and type of sounds. This ability affects both musicality and the phonological awareness needed for speech and reading.

Neuroscientific research shows that music is correlated with the executive functions of attention and memory (Cheung et al., 2017; Winner et al., 2013). The concentration required to learn a musical instrument may improve a person's general ability to focus attention and concentrate. Shahin, Roberts, Chau, Trainor, and Miller (2008) found that children who had had at least a year of music lessons had enhanced gamma-band activity (GBA), a neural response associated with attention, learning, and memory. The authors conclude that this response is neuroplastic, meaning the children's brains were more able to reorganize by forming new connections between brain cells. Kraus and Chandrasekaran (2010) state, "music training results in structural and functional biological changes throughout our lifetimes. Such neuroplasticity not only benefits music processing but also percolates to other domains" (p. 604). A limited period of childhood music lessons (around 3 years) has been found to alter the nervous system and these neural changes persist in adulthood after auditory training has ceased (Skoe & Kraus, 2012).

Musical stimuli are processed in the same centers of the brain associated with pleasure, and therefore induce optimal levels of arousal (not too high or too low) for increased learning (Hodges & Sebald, 2011). A second-grade teacher who incorporates singing into her lessons, for example, often does so out of an intuitive belief that singing a phrase that contains a new grammatical lesson will help the children retain the knowledge. Research is now proving this teacher's instincts to be correct: singing engages areas of the brain involved in learning new language skills, reinforcing reproduction and helping to retain concepts learned in the classroom (Hodges & Sebald, 2011). Engaging in sing-song vocalizations or verbalizations engages more areas of the brain, increasing connectivity and engagement.

Music is at the forefront of research into neurogenesis and neuroplasticity, as it is a modality that not only helps the brain heal from trauma and regulate internal systems (Berkowitz, 2016), but also activates the brain's ability to reroute damaged neural circuits and regain abilities thought to be lost (Taylor, 2010). We are only beginning to understand how music can create new neural networks in damaged or underdeveloped areas. People who have suffered strokes relearn how to speak through playing an instrument (Grau-Sánchez, Ramos, Duarte, Särkämö, & Rodríguez-Fornells, 2017), and people with Parkinson's disease regain muscle strength by vocalizing and singing (Fogg-Rogers et al., 2016). The brain is seemingly endless in its ability to rewire broken or damaged connections, but it needs prompting, something to help it create these new pathways (Karmonik et al., 2016). Music fulfills this need.

By reaching all areas of a child's neurological circuits, music serves as an integrative force. It not only parallels physical, emotional, and cognitive development in children, it holds the power to move them beyond barriers of disability, trauma, and atypical maturation (Kraus, Hornickel, Strait, Slater, & Thompson, 2014). Music taps into a natural source of inspiration and allows neural connections to be made that would otherwise not be possible. For example, a child who is being taught to overcome a stutter may, as part of his therapy, undergo endless repetitions of short verbal phrases. Yet add a simple rhythmic beat to the phrase and suddenly the child, seemingly without effort, can speak the phrase. Firmly connecting the beat to the phrase helps the child gain confidence in his ability to speak, and by gradually reducing the intensity of the beat the child masters the phrase with ever more accuracy. Singing phrases is also another way to help children say what is difficult for them to express, whether for developmental or emotional reasons. The brain hears a phrase that is sung differently than a phrase that is spoken, and by engaging the child's natural propensity for melody and rhythm, something that is otherwise difficult to speak becomes a song the child is eager to sing. When singing a phrase that has emotional power, the amygdala is engaged, the limbic system responds, deeper breathing is activated, and dopamine is released into the body. The child feels good, even when singing about a difficult issue or memory.

Table 4.1 summarizes findings from both behavioral and neurological research regarding the benefits of music.

Participating in Music

Human beings come into this world with innate capacities to intuit and understand melodies, rhythms, and harmonies. Even as infants we respond to subtle changes in music. It is well-known that children learn through *doing*, that is, through acting on their environment and discovering the consequences (Bartholomew, Jowers, Errisuriz, Vaughn, & Roberts, 2017). Play a piece of lively music and most children will be up dancing and singing in no time! Make instruments available and they will spontaneously gravitate to exploring how to make sounds on them. Fine and gross motor skills are refined through movement to music and through instrumental playing. Emotional development can be encouraged through role playing in musical dramas, and through self-expression in singing or playing instruments. A vast range of emotional experience is possible through music; different kinds of music elicit different moods and degrees of intensity. Having successful experiences in music boosts self-esteem (Elvers, Fischinger, & Steffens, 2017). Cognitively, songs can reinforce concepts and vocabulary. Through music, children experience form and order, from the simple to the complex (Beer, 2011).

Musicking is a word coined by Small (1998), who argued that music is not a noun or object, but rather a verb or activity. "Musicking" is a process that involves listening, singing, playing an instrument, composing, and/or dancing. Just as we are cooking when we cook, or we are

TABLE 4.1. Known Benefits of Music

Cognitive	
Improves academic achievement	Patel (2017); Young et al. (2013)
Increases IQ	Winner et al. (2013)
Improves reading skills	Carpentier et al. (2016)
Increases mathematical skills	Patel (2017)
Heightens visual–spatial skills	Patel (2017)
Strengthens executive functions of attention and memory	Cheung et al. (2017); Standley (2002); Taylor (2010)
Promotes long-lasting improvements in cognitive abilities	Schellenberg (2005)
Improves spatial–temporal reasoning	Hallam (2016); Hetland & Winner (2004); Rauscher et al. (1997)
Language development	
Increases verbal intelligence	Hallam (2016); Moreno et al. (2011)
Enriches early childhood language development	Lorenzo et al. (2014)
Enhances sensitivity to emotions conveyed by speech prosody	Thompson et al. (2004)
Improves listening skills, auditory discrimination, and perception of speech sounds	Carpentier et al. (2016); Moreno et al. (2009); Trainor et al. (2003)
Helps people with neurological damage relearn language skills	Grau-Sánchez et al. (2017); Fogg-Rogers et al. (2016)
Social–emotional	
Increases creativity	Berkowitz (2016); Passanisi et al. (2015)
Improves interpersonal relationships with peers	Passanisi et al. (2015); Lonie (2010)
Enhances parent–child relationships	Hallam (2016); Lonie (2010)
Boosts self-esteem	Elvers et al. (2018)

talking when we talk, we are musicking when we make music. To musick is to be actively involved with sounds and relationships with other people and the natural world. This idea serves to broaden our understanding of what happens when a child is "doing" music. Music "is something we *do*, and this is an *informed* doing, embodying a specific form of knowledge" (Aigen, 2014, p. 21).

The capacity to find meaning in musical experience exists in all people, regardless of disability or challenge. It is the part of us that innately responds to music, and finds it meaningful and engaging, Children are naturally drawn to music and have a love for listening and playing. Nordoff and Robbins (2007) found participating in music making with a child stimulates responses not otherwise as easily accessed. Young children instinctively engage in musical experiences, allowing for strengths in communication and socialization to surface.

How a child plays music reveals a great deal about him: a child whose drum beating is scattered and chaotic may have an inner life characterized by disorder and confusion. In contrast, a child who can maintain a steady pulse in time with the music and is flexible with dynamics is more

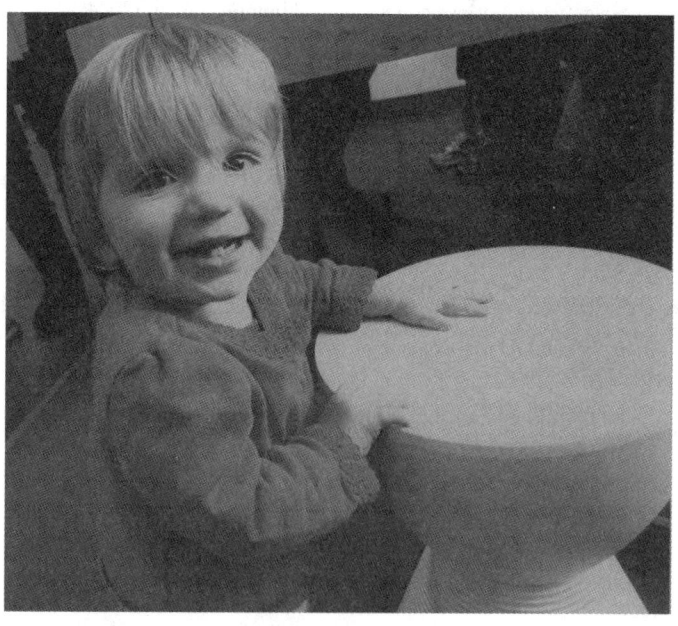

Toddler at drum

likely to be well grounded and organized perceptually and neurologically (Gaston, 1968). Knowing how musical impulses reflect the child's emotional state and ability to organize himself aids a psychotherapist in assessing and effectively treating the child.

Participation in music is a multisensory experience—our visual, tactile, and auditory systems are stimulated simultaneously. When beating a drum, for example, we *see* the mallet and the drum; we *feel* the mallet in our hand and the contact it makes with the drumhead as we raise and lower our arm to play; and we *hear* the sound the drum produces along with the accompanying music. This seemingly simple act of beating a drum involves motor planning, gross motor skills, auditory processing (knowing when to play), and sensory integration. If both hands are used, then coordination of the left and right sides of the body is also involved. Balance and our proprioceptive sense, or knowing where we are in space, come into play as well.

With any music activity, things are happening on many levels simultaneously. Take the example of a song and group instrumental activity in which the children, seated in a circle, place single drum beats at the ends of phrases. The leader sings the song while holding and offering a small hand drum to each child in turn for them to play. Going around the circle creates a sense of expectation and increases attentiveness. If the leader decides to present the drum in random order, she is introducing the element of surprise (who will be next?). The experience becomes even more exciting for the children and fosters a sense of comradery among them as well as with the leader. The clear, repetitive musical form—the phrase with a space at the end for the drum beat—helps each child perceive and process what he is hearing (executive functioning and cognition), notice what others are doing (socialization), and focus on the activity (attention span and impulse control). Further, motor planning and coordination are required for him to mobilize his body to respond quickly. By filling in a single beat, the child learns the mathematical concept of 1. The social skills of turn taking and listening to others (key components of conversation) are reinforced. Impulse control is strengthened as the child waits for the place in the music where his response is needed. The lyrics of the song, which may describe the action or have meaning for the child, aid in language acquisition and comprehension. By experiencing pleasure in the music and in his participation, the child develops positive feelings about himself, his peers, and his community. Important to note here is the role of repetition, which is acknowledged to be an important element of musical development. Research indicates the repetition involved with learning musical forms and ways of playing correlates to language development (Patel & Morgan, 2017). Repetition also leads to increased mastery and self-confidence (Nordoff & Robbins, 2007).

Engaging in music experiences changes how a child thinks about and responds to his environment. It can also shape interactions when used intentionally and with care. Similar to play therapy, music can act as a third force in the therapy room, offering the child an alternative to interacting directly with the therapist (Crenshaw, Brooks, & Goldstein, 2015). A child who is unwilling to make eye contact will often focus intently on playing an instrument. Music can serve as a form of parallel play and also as the psychological space between child and therapist, binding them together in a shared place of mutual engagement (Levinge, 2015).

Models of Musical Development in Young Children

Various models of child development serve as a guide to help understand the cognitive, physical, and social–emotional functioning level of clients. In what areas is the child on target developmentally? In what areas is he advanced or behind what is expected of a child his age? This understanding, in turn, helps us identify areas of need and informs interventions. Models of development have moved from an emphasis on intrapsychic processes, or a one-person psychology, to a two-person psychology that focuses on interpersonal and intersubjective processes (Stern, 2008). Musical interaction, which is often nonverbal and depends on a child's innate ability to communicate, may be the most appropriate intervention for the development of early relationships, learning to recognize emotions, and other skills (Briggs, 2015).

Likewise, when using music with children, it is helpful to know what is typical of children at different ages and stages of development. Developmental models are useful clinically in both the assessment and the treatment process (Briggs, 1991, 2015). Briggs and Bruscia (1985) developed a comprehensive and systematic model for understanding musical development that integrates models of child development. Just as there are developmental phases in the acquisition of language, cognition, social skills, and other areas, there are distinct phases of musical development. Briggs (1991) identified four phases in the first 6 years of life. For each phase, she described musical milestones in three areas: auditory, vocal/

tonal, and rhythmic. The following is a brief summary of Briggs's four phases of musical development.

- *The reflex phase (ages birth to 9 months).* During this first phase, children actively take in sensory information around them while using their own vocal and rhythmic skills to communicate their needs to their caregivers. For example, a typically developing 6-month-old infant vocalizes frequently, responds to his environment and people around him, and also uses his voice to communicate his needs. At this age an infant is able to search for a musical source, can vocally match pitches sung to him, and moves to music with his whole body. During this phase, a parent or therapist might engage the infant in vocal play by coming in close proximity and making a variety of cooing, shhh, and other soothing sounds. Quiet singing helps calm an infant who is distressed. Rocking an infant or moving his limbs in time to music gives him a rhythmic experience that helps him regulate and organize himself.

- *The intention phase (ages 9 to 18 months).* During this period, the child begins the process of separation-individuation and starts to develop a concept of himself as a separate being. In this phase the child localizes sound sources, moves to music with separate body parts, recognizes familiar songs, and engages in musical babbling, making song-like or speech-like sounds using repeated syllables with vowels and consonants, such as "ba-ba-ba." This kind of babbling has a recognizable sing-song melody and resembles real language, for young children intuitively pick up the inflections of the speech that they hear. When we work with young children, making these types of vocalizations is a way to meet them developmentally and work with them at their linguistic and cognitive level. Engage the baby in vocal play that includes vocal slides (sliding from one pitch to another, like the sound of a siren) and repeated consonant–vowel syllables. Bounce the baby on your lap and move together along with the beat of the music or a song. Play movement games that use separate body parts (clapping hands, moving arms up and down, stamping feet). Repeat singing songs that the child knows and add some new ones.

- *The control phase (ages 18 to 36 months).* This third phase is dominated by the struggle to control impulses and to feel in control of one's environment. The child enjoys listening to music quietly for several minutes and develops improved pitch perception and pitch accuracy. Children at this age love to sing, though their singing range is still narrow, and they gradually shift from musical babbling to more recognizable singing of melodies. As the child develops better motor control, he shows an increase in variety of movements to music. During this phase, children enjoy vigorous music that has strong, pounding rhythms. Encourage the child to join you in singing favorite songs. Provide opportunities for the child to choose actions in movement games and to make choices about how and what instrument to play. For a therapist treating a child older than 3 years who has attachment issues or suffers from the results of a trauma, reverting to the salient features of this stage can be a healthy way to engage them and stimulate development. Singing simple melodies of children's songs and moving to music that has a strong beat, for example, gives them a means to reassert a sense of internal control.

- *The integration phase (3 to 6 years of age).* By the end of this fourth phase, children have completed the separation-individuation process and the personality becomes more formed. Listening skills and pitch perception improve significantly, and children learn to discriminate loud and soft sounds. They sing both spontaneous songs and learned songs with increasing pitch accuracy. At this age, children delight in making up repetitive little songs or chants with original lyrics, often about themselves, or rhymes with nonsense words. When my (J. C. B.'s) son was 4 years old, he would go around the house singing, "Poopsie pies are great, I can't believe I ate, POOPSIE PIES!" He thought it was wonderfully funny, though we never were able to ascertain what, exactly, poopsie pies were. Rhythmically, children show improvement in eye–hand coordination, organization of rhythmic behaviors (e.g., beating rhythmic patterns), and speed and range of movements. At around age 5, children are still sorting out musical concepts and may confuse loud with fast, and soft with slow. As they get older they acquire the ability to internalize a pulse, or feel the beat of the music inside the body whether or not the music is playing. At this stage, children need experience with a widening range of music, rhythms, and songs. As therapists, we can nurture their creativity by providing musical materials and an attitude of acceptance and encouragement.

Schwartz (2008), building on the work of Briggs, Bruscia, and others, outlines typical musical responses at different ages. She describes five developmental levels—*awareness, trust, independence, control,* and *responsibility*—and the behaviors a child would commonly display at each of these levels with respect to singing, playing, music movement, and musical understandings (which includes listening). For each level she lists corresponding goals and objectives, as well as possible strategies and interventions to help children reach these developmental goals. Schwartz (2008) also discusses various diagnoses and how they might impact musical development.

Guilmartin and Levinowitz (2008) founded Music Together, a program for children ages birth–7 years and their families based on research in both music and child development. The overriding aim of Music Together is to help children become musically competent through developmentally appropriate musical experiences with caring adults. The program is based on the belief that all children are musical and thus have the potential to achieve tonal and rhythmic competence. They define basic music competence as audiation (the ability to hear music in your head when it is not physically present), the ability to sing in tune, and rhythmic expression through accurate movement.

There is a critical period—up to age 5—when a child's musical aptitude is most readily influenced by the environment (Guilmartin & Levinowitz, 2008). Based on their observations of young children, they delineate the tonal and rhythmic skills that develop at different ages, given an enriched musical environment. For example, a child progresses from sustaining single pitches to filling in ends of song phrases to singing entire songs in tune. Rhythmically, a child shifts from expressing his own internal rhythm to moving or singing along with the beat of the music to being able to maintain a correct tempo or rhythmic pattern when there is no external music. Most children advance through these various stages in a predictable order, and each child proceeds at his own pace. Table 4.2 outlines several developmental processes related to music as well as suggestions for appropriate strategies.

While it is helpful to know how musical skills unfold in children, it is also important to view these various models of musical development in a broad context. A child's musical development is a part of his overall development right through adulthood. As discussed in Chapter 3, a humanistic approach to child development (DeRobertis, 2008) emphasizes a holistic perspective that recognizes the uniqueness of each child and is situated in an individual's historical and cultural context. DeRobertis views growth as an active, not passive, process, one that "values an understanding of healthy development" (2008, p. 8). Music is a pursuit that is naturally enriching for children and brings together physical, emotional, and social processes that will have an impact on the life span and unique identity of that individual.

TABLE 4.2. Musical Development

Basic abilities	Strategies/interventions
Ages birth–5 months	
• Hearing begins to develop. • Cries around one central pitch. • At 2 months, has fixed attention when sung to. • At 3 months, becomes calm when quiet music is played. • Distinguishes between two pitches and two timbres. • Makes "coo" sounds and reacts to others' sounds. • Makes involuntary, irregular movements in response to a musical stimulus.	• Engage in vocal play (provided infant is stable), using *coo, shhuu*, and other sounds typical of a mother comforting a child. • Sing lullabies and other calming songs. • Rock the infant to quiet music. • Use touch along with music to stimulate sensory response. • Move infant's limbs rhythmically in time to music.
Ages 6–9 months	
• Searches for music source. • Increases frequency and variety of vocalizations. • Vocally matches pitches sung to them. • Moves to music with whole body.	• Move sources of music around the room. • Continue to engage in vocal play using a variety of consonant/vowel syllables. • Gently bounce baby on your lap to rhythmic chants and songs.
Ages 9–12 months	
• Vocal range increases but child is unable to control pitches. • Localizes sound sources. • Recognizes familiar songs. • Gains more muscle control and moves to a musical stimulus.	• Engage in vocal play using vocal slides and repeated syllables. • Create silly sounds that reflect the child's activities or movements. • Bounce and move together to music. • Sing familiar songs, with lots of repetition.
Ages 12–24 months	
• Babbles musically in a sing-song, repetitive vocal style. • Starts to sing endings and beginnings of song phrases. • Has more accurate pitch perception and sings recognizable pitches.	• Continue to engage in reciprocal vocal play. • Sing songs and encourage the child to sing along with you; allow the child to fill in endings of phrases. • Provide music with a simple rhythmic beat for the child to move to.

(continued)

TABLE 4.2. *(continued)*

Basic abilities	Strategies/interventions

Ages 12–24 months *(continued)*

- Follows the song's melodic contour when singing.
- Moves to music with separate body parts.
- Sustains repeated movements at a consistent tempo.
- At 18 months, prefers to move to music with a partner/other.

- Play movement games that use separate body parts (clapping hands, stamping feet).
- Offer opportunities to make choices of what and how to play.

Ages 2–3 years

- Listens to music quietly for several minutes.
- Shows great interest in singing and remembers lyrics, but recognizes only few words of a song.
- Uses singing voice in a more sustained fashion.
- Pitch perception continues to improve.
- Shows increase in variety of movements to music.
- Demonstrates large increase in rhythmic/motor control, but movements do not necessarily coincide with the music's beat.
- Enjoys strong pounding and banging rhythms.

- Listen to softer, slower pieces of music with the child.
- Sing songs of all kinds.
- Provide age-appropriate recorded music.
- Engage in movement games that use more variety of movements (wiggling fingers, rolling hands, shrugging shoulders).
- Encourage dancing to music.
- Play with musical starts and stops.
- Provide opportunities for rhythmic activities (e.g., beating a drum).

Ages 3–4 years

- Sings spontaneous songs using short phrases; continues to sing after the musical stimulus has ended.
- Sings parts of a song correctly.
- Pitch perception continues to become more accurate.
- Can discriminate "loud."
- Coordinates singing and moving simultaneously.
- Can do learned movement to music.
- Shows steady improvement in eye–hand coordination, and speed and range of movements.

- Make up songs about the child's likes and dislikes; these can be set to familiar melodies.
- Engage in rhythmic games, for example, by taking turns initiating and imitating rhythmic patterns on a drum.
- Engage the child in large motor movements to music (marching, jumping, galloping).
- Engage the child in songs that have movement sequences ("Where Is Thumbkin?", "This Old Man").
- Provide instruments for the child to explore that require fine-hand coordination (e.g., xylophone).

(continued)

TABLE 4.2. *(continued)*

Basic abilities	Strategies/interventions
Ages 4–6 years	
• Recognizes familiar songs consistently. • Sings with lyrics, melody, rhythm, phrasing, and pulse. • Shows large growth in song repertoire. • Understands musical concepts (high/low, loud/soft, fast/slow) but cannot describe or demonstrate them. • Coordinates upper and lower body to the beat with rhythmic accuracy. • Continues to show improvement in eye–hand coordination, and speed and range of movements.	• Introduce new songs. • Provide experiences in the polarities of musical elements (high/low, loud/soft, fast/slow). • Provide rhythmic experiences with more complex meters. • Continue to provide a variety of instruments for the child to explore that require fine-hand coordination (xylophone, resonator bells).
Ages 6 years and older	
• Sings an entire song correctly and in tune. • Synchronizes movements to the beat of the music. • Can begin to demonstrate musical concepts (high/low, loud/soft, fast/slow). • Shows large increase in listening skills. • Continues to show improvement in eye–hand coordination, and speed and range of movements.	• Expose the child to a variety of music, including recorded music and live concerts. • Teach the child simple musical parts (how to play a simple melody or maintain a rhythmic pattern on a drum). • Experiment with ranges of dynamics and tempos. • Allow opportunities for music making with peers.

MUSIC AND ADOLESCENCE

One of the vital tasks of adolescence is establishing one's own identity separate from that of the family (Hadiwijaya, Klimstra, Vermunt, Branje, & Meeus, 2017). This is accomplished in part by challenging adult norms and expectations and discovering the consequences. The peer group assumes primary importance during these years, and the music a teen shares with his friends becomes laden with meaning. This music may fall well outside the preference of a therapist, yet when making music with adolescents, the therapist must show respect for their preferred music, even if she does not like or understand it. We suspect that most people still love the music of their teenage years long after those years have passed. We know that patients in nursing homes often respond to the music of their youth when nothing else seems to reach them—they may sing along to older, familiar songs even when they no longer have access to speech.

In our work with adolescents we have experienced many times a spontaneous responsiveness to music that overrides the teen's natural inclination to be resistant or closed off to adult interactions. Becoming engaged in music pursuits or discussions about music is a way to address therapeutic issues. For example, a teen in an inpatient psychiatric facility would not speak directly to his counselor about any emotional issues or difficulties he had relating to others. In a group therapy session, the counselor suggested that each member choose a song for the group to listen to with the proviso the song would not have violent or misogynistic lyrics. The teen was eager to select a song and afterward talked about how it represented the singer's anger at the world and how he felt misunderstood. This young man did not have to say, "I feel angry," but his passion in talking about the song was strong. It opened a door for the therapist to engage the entire group in a discussion about anger.

At the same time, it is important for therapists using music with teens to have some understanding of the potentially negative effects music can have and be alert to when it is time to disengage from a music experience with a client. Saarikallio and Erkkilä (2007) found that if adolescents happened to start listening to a song that they associated with difficult memories, they often felt worse for it. A sensitive and attuned psychotherapist can work with a child or teen's natural desire to listen to songs that somehow reflect their private emotional landscape, but may need to identify when this desire becomes overwhelming or toxic in some way. Older children may have internalized judgments or fears of not being good enough, so musical experiences must be presented with careful consideration for the client's sensitivities, history, and preferences. Overall, tapping into this sometimes unpredictable world can yield therapeutic benefits as, for some children and teenagers, music is a force that helps them survive. As Toni, a teen participant in the study, said,

> [Music] is life . . . you start living when there's music. Because to live without music, there would be nothing . . . without music there would be no feelings in life, in a way. It is so that . . . you, like, visit this world, and it's the sugar on the top. (in Saarikallio & Erkkilä, 2007, p. 97)

MUSIC AND EMOTIONS

Western music is typically played in either a major or minor key, which may evoke associations of feeling happy or sad. The connections between the music we hear and what we feel are strong and sometimes surprising. It is known that playing fast music will speed up a person's heart rate, and calm music can lower blood pressure, prompt us to breathe more deeply, and decrease levels of chemicals in our body that cause stress (Taylor, 2010). Recent studies, however, also show that while people are drawn to happy-sounding music when they feel happy, they are also attracted to sad music when they feel happy: it is soothing and brings a sense of peace. Listening to sad music actually helps people feel better (Garrido, 2009; Van den Tol & Edwards, 2013).

Charles Schulz, the creator of the *Peanuts* comic strip, once said, "Happiness is a sad song" (1967). Music that has a mournful sound brings comfort (Vuokoski & Eerola, 2017; Vuoskoski, Thompson, McIlwain, & Eerola, 2012). This apparent contradiction between what we feel and what we choose to listen to has fascinated psychologists and musicologists for many years. There is growing interest in research and development of theories of emotion in psychology; studies show that when people feel happy they often seek out sad music to reinforce the feeling (Plamper, 2015), for music is multidimensional and reflects the complexity of our emotional states. It is not a stretch to say that people choose to listen to sad music to help them feel happier, and also when they are happy and seeking to feel a greater sense of peace (Kawakami, Furukawa, Katahira, & Okanoya, 2013; Saarikallio & Erkkilä, 2007). Finding ways to incorporate music into psychotherapy with children can support their ability to hold contradictions, such as: I can feel angry but keep calm; I can feel happy but still relate to my friend who is feeling sad.

One study had an interesting implication for children learning to cope with their emotions (Vuoskoski et al., 2012). The authors found "openness to experience and empathy were associated with a liking for sad music and with the intensity of emotional responses induced by sad music" (Vuoskoski et al., 2012, p. 311). For children with varying issues, having empathy and remaining open to experiences are important pieces of social interaction. Listening to favorite songs can be a safe way to retrieve memories, feel more connected to people around you, experience a lift in mood, or simply be distracted from difficult events or thoughts (Van den Tol & Edwards, 2011). Think about how, after a tough day at school or work, you might go home and put on some of your favorite music to listen to. It can brighten your mood, and feeling better can help to keep problems in perspective.

The primary reason we listen to and play music is to have an emotional experience (Saarikallio & Erkkilä, 2007). Identifying songs and listening to them is something a psychotherapist without much training in music could potentially do in her practice, yet, as discussed above, we caution therapists to be vigilant about possible unanticipated responses.

CULTURAL LENS

The development of a child's musical tastes is directly shaped by the cultural environment into which he is born. Children in all cultures learn the music unique to that culture. Songs or chants are often passed down orally, and as children participate in rituals and in the daily life of their families and communities, the sounds of their culture become part of their heritage. Through folk songs, children learn about societal norms and expectations, gain historical and mythological knowledge, and acquire needed information and skills to participate successfully in their cultural milieu (Seri & Gilboa, 2017). The songs are meant to both entertain and instruct all ages (Glen, 2017). It is a relatively modern idea to have composers writing and performing songs specifically for children. Children's music is now an enormous industry, and there are numerous resources available on the Internet for ideas for finding culturally appropriate musical songs, games, and interventions.

Identifying which formats and songs are a good fit for a specific clinical situation takes thought and planning. Suggestions for doing this include talking with parents about what songs their child responds to or likes to sing or dance to, and bringing in music suited to the child's developmental age. Music, when brought into therapy, can support a child's expression and serve as a natural way to ensure the client's cultural heritage is included in treatment. It may also serve as a barrier to treatment or lead to unexpected consequences as shown in the case example below.

VIGNETTE

Seiichi was a 10-year-old boy who was referred to Sheree, a play therapist. Seiichi had been acting out at home and at school and his parents were anxious to help him become, "the happy, normal little boy he'd always been." When Sheree first spoke with Seiichi's mother, Hidemi, she learned that Hidemi spoke English as a second language, with Japanese being her first language. Hidemi said she was embarrassed to ask for help, but school officials had strongly recommended she seek help for Seiichi. Sheree recognized that Hidemi might be experiencing a feeling of shame that could be rooted in a cultural belief that one should not air troubles to anyone outside of the family. She knew that in the collectivistic culture of Japan, family honor may be valued above individual need. She was quick to reassure Hidemi that sometimes children need help, and also that their work would be kept strictly confidential. Hidemi seemed relieved and told Sheree that Seichii had been having problems ever since they had returned from Japan after her father's funeral there. Seiichi had spent several summers in Japan at his grandparents' home and had become close with his grandfather.

In reflecting on her conversation with Hidemi, Sheree felt Seichi might be experiencing a confused grief response. The cultural norms for death and the rituals surrounding it are different in Japan and Seichii might have been having trouble reconciling his teachers' concern about how he was feeling following the loss of his grandfather with his belief that he should not be talking about it. Sheree wondered if he was caught between two worlds. She also felt confident she could help him. On a personal level, Sheree felt an affinity with the religious tenets of Buddhism and had placed a small statue of a Buddha and a Tibetan singing bowl in the therapy room. She felt the placement of these objects reflected her personal philosophy of therapy as an endeavor that reaches across internal and external borders, and demonstrated a sense of inclusivity and warmth. She also had a ritual of gently ringing the singing bowl right before she welcomed children into the therapy room.

The first time she met Seiichi she rang the singing bowl, then greeted him in the waiting room and invited him into the therapy room. He glared at her but got up and followed her when he was admonished by his mother: "Go! Go!" Once in the room, Sheree began to identify some of the things that he could play with: a sand tray, a tubano drum, puppets, action figures, drawing materials, and clay. He looked around the room and appeared to be nervous, walking quickly and shaking his hands. He went over to the puppets and explored the various characters and animals represented. He then picked up several of the figurines, choosing an older man. He laid the man down on his back and said "You're dead! Don't get up! I don't see you!" His voice did not sound angry when he said this, but it was forceful. He covered the man with a tissue and then went back to playing with the puppets. Sheree talked with Seiichi about the puppets he liked, their names and ages, and was surprised at how readily he let her into his play world. She sensed that the figurine of the older man might symbolize his grandfather but did not want to push him on this. At the end of the session she asked Seiichi, "Should we leave the man covered up, or should we uncover him before you leave?" He replied, "No, leave him covered." Sheree agreed, and they talked for a few moments about what they could do together next week.

Afterward, Sheree called Hidemi to review the session, and Hidemi said, "I think I might know what happened. When we were waiting in the room for therapy to begin, Seiichi and I heard you ring the singing bowl. I'm not sure if you know this, but the bowl is part of the funeral ritual in Japan. The last time Seiichi heard this played was at my father's funeral." Sheree paused, not yet sure what to make of this information. She asked Hidemi, "Do you think him hearing the bowl at therapy had an effect?" Hidemi replied, "Yes, I do. When we heard it we looked at each other, so surprised. He asked me, 'Mommy, is someone else dying?' I told him no, you were playing it as part of your own practice. When you came out to us to bring him into therapy, I had to encourage him to go."

Sheree told Hidemi how openly Seiichi had responded, showing no signs of anger during the session. Hidemi felt this may have been because he was remembering his grandfather and the funeral, and perhaps was feeling sad. Sheree realized the session could have gone in a different direction: Seiichi could have reacted to the sound of the singing bowl with intense grief, anger, or by shutting down emotionally. She had had no idea that the bowl was part of the funeral ritual in Japan, and knew she had to be more careful in using this instrument. She gave a lot of thought as to whether to use the bowl again next week before Seiichi came into the room. She decided that his willingness to engage in talking and playing with her reflected his ability to tolerate his feelings of grief, and that he might be expecting to hear the sound again next week. To take it away would be to make something else disappear, just as his grandfather had disappeared from his life.

When Seiichi and his mother next arrived, Sheree played the bowl before welcoming him into the room, then waited a few seconds before greeting him. She wanted to give him time to process the sound before coming into the therapy room. This time he needed no prompting, and as soon as he entered the room he looked to see if the figurine was still covered by the tissue. Sheree had carefully reconstructed the placement of the figurine to match where it was last session, and upon seeing it Seiichi smiled and said softly, "He is still here." Sheree asked him who the figure was, and he responded that it was his grandfather. From there he shared details about the long flight to Japan, seeing his relatives, and how different things were there. She asked him if he could show her, either through the puppets or the figurines, who the people were and how they acted. He agreed and showed Sheree some of what he had experienced while in Japan.

Over a period of a few weeks, Seiichi shared more about his grandfather. He processed his grief in a variety of ways, using music, puppetry, and sand play. Reports from school and home indicated his outbursts were decreasing, and after 11 sessions he told Sheree he wanted to play soccer, but practice was at the same time as his meetings with her. Sheree and Hidemi agreed that his time in therapy had come to a close. Hidemi was relieved her child was feeling better, and she was also more able to talk with him about his grandfather and share some memories with him.

When she wrote up her final notes, Sheree reflected on the power of the one sound, the ringing of the bowl, and how it had affected Sheiichi emotionally more than any words could have. She discontinued her practice of ringing the bowl before sessions but kept it handy in case she had a future situation which might warrant its use.

SUMMARY

Music has its own developmental progression, parallel to and intersecting with a child's physical, cognitive, social, and emotional development. Many children seen for therapy experience a lapse or delay in one area, and music can be helpful in working on these domains from a position of strength and ability. With its global effect, music holds the potential to strengthen lagging areas by accessing those that the child naturally responds to and feels confident in.

RECOMMENDATIONS FOR PRACTICE

When deciding on strategies and activities, it is important to consider the child's developmental level with respect to the levels of musical development described above; a child may be delayed or advanced for his chronological age. With this thought in mind, it is also advisable that interventions be reasonably age-appropriate. For example, when helping an adolescent with a speech delay you might choose to work within the context of a current pop song rather than an early childhood song such as "The Wheels on the Bus."

- Moving to music engages a child's neurological, motor, and self-expressive capabilities. Suggestions for helping a child develop skills in these areas include dancing freely to various kinds of music and dancing with scarves. Choosing music from cultures other than the one the child is associated with can evoke spontaneous movements, for example, playing Bollywood songs for North American children.
- Creating mini-musical dramas is a highly pleasurable way for children to problem-solve, be creative, and interact with each other. Take one of the child's favorite stories and find a piece of music that fits part of it (classical music works well here, for it does not have words to distract the child), and retell the story using dramatic voices and actions. Have the child help voice the characters and choose movements that suit the music. One idea is to take a popular story such as *Goodnight Moon* (Brown, 2007) and select instruments to represent the various characters.
- With a child who has difficulty expressing himself through spoken words due to speech or developmental delays, it is helpful to remember how powerfully music affects various speech and language centers in the brain. Connecting with the rhythmic nature of speech can prompt his engagement, and putting the speech patterns into musical sound makes this a natural and pleasurable interaction.
  - Choose a phrase with which you think the child is familiar, and, with some work, could master. For the purpose of this recommendation, let's choose "*I want milk.*"
  - First speak the phrase and ask the child to repeat it; this gives you a baseline of how the child says the words. Listen carefully for where the child puts the stressed syllables.
  - Play the phrase on a small drum using your hand just as you hear it, then hold the drum out to the child to repeat the phrase. Go back and forth two or three times.
  - Add a "ta" sound to replace the syllables. For example, for "I want MILK!" say "ta ta TA" in the rhythm and speed the child originally spoke the phrase. Continue adding the drum beat for reinforcement, and go back and forth several times, taking turns with the client.

- This may be a good time to stop so that the child does not become overwhelmed or overstimulated. Take a break and go to another exercise for a while or wait until the next session to come back to this exercise. Giving the child time and space to integrate the levels of learning is important.
- When you come back to it, repeat the first three steps. Next, slow the phrase down using the "ta" sound. Once the child is able to slow the phrase down, add the words back in, continuing to use the drum beat to keep a sense of continuity and support.
- Repeat all steps, moving between them as called for.
• With adolescents, share playlists. Listen to each other's music and talk about each other's responses.

Working with Groups

When working with a group of young children, fostering individual expression while strengthening social awareness is possible through group exercises. With a group, for example, of 5-year-old children who have communication and social development delays, simply adding a beat to the end of song phrases and having them take turns adding the special beat can create a sense of enthusiasm, engagement, and awareness of each other.

• Prepare by having a triangle with striker and a small hand drum in a bag behind your chair or area. Have the children seated in a semicircle, either in chairs or on carpet squares. Choose a familiar song such as "Baa, Baa, Black Sheep" (to the tune of the "The ABC Song") and sing it through two or three times with the children.
• With some sense of anticipation, bring out the bag of instruments and see if the children can guess what is inside.
• Take out the triangle and striker, and while you hold the triangle, give each child a turn to hold the striker and briefly play the triangle.
• Sing the song through again, this time with you modeling how to play the triangle at the end of each phrase, pausing the song to hear the instrument sound.
• Either choose a child to go first whom you know might be successful in doing this exercise or ask the children who wants to go first.

- With a sense of ceremony, hand the triangle and striker to the child, have him play it once, and then ask if the other children are ready to sing.
- Sing the song, creating space at the end of each phrase for the triangle to be heard.
- Either choose another child to take the triangle or ask for a volunteer again and repeat the previous steps.
- If you think a slight change will help keep the children's attention, you can change the song to "The ABC Song" or "Twinkle, Twinkle, Little Star" (both have the same melody as "Baa, Baa, Black Sheep"), or replace the triangle with another instrument.
- If the children are able to continue, have two children play together at the ends of phrases, one with the triangle and one with the hand drum.
- For another layer of complexity, add different instruments for each phrase ending and have the children switch instruments. Close the exercise when you feel their attention is beginning to wane.
- For children who have delays, tailoring music experiences to fit their developmental age can be done by shifting techniques and choices. A 6-year-old child who has Down syndrome may respond better to finger plays such as "The Itsy Bitsy Spider" or "Where Is Thumbkin?" than to an activity that is cognitively more complex, such as creating new lyrics to a familiar song.

CHAPTER 5

Attachment and Attunement in Interpersonal Relationships

> We humans interact with one another at great speed, synchronizing with subtle rhythms of exchange. Our bodies express the impulses of our minds, and we react immediately to one another's expressions. Music makes this into sound that appeals directly to the inner sense of acting and feeling. This is a level of meaning where words may be superfluous.
> —Trevarthen (1997, p. x)

The concept of attachment refers to the enduring emotional connection between two people that "draws on humans' innate tendency to form bonds with others" (Gazzaniga, 2018, p. 347). In theories of child development, attachment is specific to the trusting and loving relationship a baby forms with his or her caregiver (Bowlby, 2005; Mitchell, 1988). The process of attachment begins before birth—in utero, the fetus hears the timbre and inflections of its mother's voice. The newborn can distinguish his mother's voice from that of other women's voices, and the preference for his mother's voice may play a role in initiating mother–infant bonding (DeCasper & Fifer, 1980).

This chapter addresses the needs of children who did not experience healthy and sustained interactions when very young. These children are at risk for impaired social relationships as well as mental and emotional issues in later life (Bowlby, 1982; DeKlyen & Greenberg, 2016). In particular, those with attachment disorders can have difficulty successfully managing their emotions, interactions with their primary caregiver may be fraught with tension, and children may become unresponsive or even rejecting of attempts to connect with them (Pearce, 2016).

Early intervention to support the development of secure attachment can have a profound effect as childrens' neuronal patterns and patterns of behavior are capable of being influenced and changed. Parental or caregiver involvement is now acknowledged to be a critical part of early treatment (Guralnick, 2017; Zanetti, Powell, Cooper, & Hoffman, 2011). Using music can be powerful in helping parents learn to respond more sensitively to their infants' cues and signals (Loewy, 2015; Porges, 2011). Likewise, music as part of attachment interventions can help older children reshape learned responses and behaviors and facilitate more positive interactions with their peers.

THEORIES OF ATTACHMENT AND ATTACHMENT-BASED INTERVENTIONS

Bowlby (2005), with seminal contributions from Ainsworth (1979; Ainsworth, Blehar, Waters, & Wall, 1978), is credited with developing an evolutionary theory of attachment based on the belief that children are born biologically preprogrammed to seek and form attachments with others. The four components of Bowlby's theory are proximity maintenance (wanting to be close to caregiver), separation distress (the child becomes upset when separated from caregiver), safe haven (caregiver is viewed by child as a person offering comfort and reassurance), and secure base (caregiver is the child's source of security and reliable information) (Zeifman & Hazan, 2016). A baby's most pressing need is for love and security, and healthy development depends upon whether physical and emotional needs are met during the first years of life.

According to attachment theorists (Bowlby, 2005; Mitchell, 1988; Stern, 2010), healthy attachment or bonding between a child and caregiver occurs during the first 2 years of life. Children with secure attachments grow to view others as loving and dependable, and view the world as a safe place where people can be relied upon and trusted. They see themselves as lovable and capable, and their emotional security allows them to tolerate stress (Bowlby, 2005). Building empathy and learning to have confidence in others is crucial to being able to cultivate positive interactions with others and develop a capacity for problem solving (Greene & Ablon, 2006).

When early attachment is disrupted, children may grow to see the world and other people as potentially dangerous and menacing. They can believe themselves to be unworthy of love and may experience feelings of despair and loss of control. Behavioral issues such as frequent outbursts, difficulties managing anger, isolative tendencies, and an inability to self-regulate emotions are common symptoms that manifest in children who have experienced such trauma (Birnbaum, 2013). These can have lasting effects on school performance (McLeod et al., 2017) as well as psychological and social development (Shiller, 2017; Thompson, 2016). Consequences can be felt into adolescence, when teens tend to either internalize responses triggered by stressful situations by falling into depression or anxious states, or externalize them with risk-taking behaviors or aggression (Allen & Tan, 2016).

Children need positive early experiences to support them in their exploration of the world, to help them feel confident, and to develop healthy relationships. Ainsworth (1967) has shown how the mother's parenting style and her responsiveness to her baby's needs can result in a secure attachment or conversely, an insecure, disorganized, or avoidant attachment. Securely attached babies have caregivers who are more responsive to their infants' signals and provide a secure base for them as they become familiar with their environment (Ainsworth, 1979). Given the importance of these early relationships, further research is ongoing on how to intervene with parents and caregivers who do not respond empathically to their child's needs due to their own personal histories or to struggles in their daily lives (Cassidy & Shaver, 2016; Wittkowski et al., 2018).

Attachment-based therapies focus on the psychobiological aspects of communication between caregiver and child, including their interactive speech, vocalizations and sounds, body language, and eye contact (Berlin, Zeanah, & Lieberman, 2016). In order to enhance early attachment, parents and caregivers need to recognize these communicative cues and respond in a sensitive manner. Creative arts therapies that are sensory-based (visual, kinesthetic, tactile, olfactory, and/or auditory) and primarily nonverbal in nature are particularly useful for intervening on these levels (Gil, 2015; Malchiodi, 2015).

Stewart, Whelan, and Pendleton (2014) have shown how the Circle of Security (COS) intervention can be used by play therapists to support safe and sensitive interactions within the therapy session. The COS intervention is defined as a "brief, behavioral, and insight-oriented therapeutic group approach for promoting attachment and autonomy in the parent–child relationship" (Ramsauer et al., 2014, p. 3). It employs a simple graphic to represent both the child's needs for intimate connection and autonomy, and parenting behaviors that support these needs. Stewart et al. (2014) show how the graphic can assist parents in observing a child's cues such as proximity, movement, physical contact, tone of voice, speech, and body language, and subsequently use these observations to respond to the child in a manner that is sensitive and attuned to the child's needs. Life histories and storytelling are also incorporated to retrain parents' automatic responses to their child's behaviors and orient them to times when their child might be miscuing them or behaving in a way that belies an underlying need (Powell, Cooper, Hoffman, & Marvin, 2014). To illustrate, a parent who has attachment issues himself might misinterpret his preverbal toddler's cry as being intentionally disruptive, when in reality it is a cry of pain or discomfort. When the parent responds by demanding the child stop crying, it is likely the child will intensify his cries, creating a cycle of miscues and escalating tension. Becoming more aware of their own memories and attachment histories helps parents separate their responses from the child's, and clears a path to responding sensitively and appropriately to the actual need.

This chapter shows how musical principles can be incorporated in such interventions to enhance parental attunement and develop secure attachments with their children.

POLYVAGAL THEORY

Breakthroughs in neuroscience have led to a biobehavioral understanding of why early relationships are so important and offer clinical implications for re-creating healthy attachments. Porges's polyvagal theory (2009, 2010, 2011) describes the role of the vagus nerve, part of the involuntary or autonomic nervous system, in the social engagement system (SES). The SES is a type of response that involves a combination of activation and calming. When confronted with imminent danger, a person may become hyperaroused and mobilized to act by either fighting or fleeing (known as the fight-or-flight response). Alternately, a life-threatening situation may result in hypoarousal and the individual may respond by becoming immobilized, or "freezing." When the SES is stimulated, it assists in calming the sympathetic nervous system and the fight/flight/freeze response, and helps to mitigate our response to danger and interpersonal threats (Porges, 2009, 2011).

Polyvagal theory illuminates the neurophysiological processes of human responses to emotional pressure and articulates our inherent need to feel secure, beginning in infancy. Porges's work establishes new, more effective ways of responding to stress and interacting with others and has important implications for the treatment of anxiety, depression, trauma, and autism (Porges, 2009, 2011).

Porges suggests that therapists adopt a steady, calm demeanor, and modulate their voices to be smooth and comforting in order to impart a sense of security and warmth to the child. When a therapist consistently models predictable and safe reactions, a child responds physiologically and the nervous system begins to calm down; he can move into an internal space of feeling secure and protected. Being steady in approach and contact is crucial, for "attachment patterns are built one interaction at a time" (Stewart et al., 2014, p. 38). Working with a child to create a new internal working model of confidence and security becomes possible (Zilberstein, 2014).

Porges also connects polyvagal theory directly to music and highlights the benefits of music in therapy. The area of the brain that responds to safety, risk, and danger is also one of the areas that responds to music. He notes that "music changes not only our emotive state, but also elicits changes in our physiology that parallel the feelings of anxiety, fear, panic, and pain" (Porges, 2010, p. 2). Rhythmic games or incorporating melody, such as singing requests or creating short songs about a child's likes and dislikes, generates a biobehavioral response that helps the child self-regulate and feel more safe and secure (Porges, 2011).

ENTRAINMENT

Entrainment is the process by which two people become aligned in their thoughts, movements, and emotions through physiological and vocal synchrony. It is a precursor to attunement and attachment. Mothers entrain with their infants by mimicking their vocal patterns, and young children reciprocate by echoing the speech patterns of their parents (Ko, Seidl, Cristia, Reimchen, & Soderstrom, 2016; Pickering & Garrod, 2004). This dynamic exchange is the basis for language and relational development: the ability to influence and follow the nuances of communication, both verbal and nonverbal, is a building block for children's growth.

Entrainment is both a physiological process (e.g., when heart rate entrains to a repeated, rhythmic beat) and a social one (e.g., when mass hysteria takes over a crowd of people). The neurophysiological theory of mirror neurons adds to our understanding of entrainment. "Mirror neurons" are the cluster of neurons that mediate perception and action, connecting what we see and experience around us to what we do (Koelsch, 2009). They fire both when we see someone do an action and when we ourselves do that same action and, when considered from a therapeutic point of view, offer a clinician a path to model healthy responses to situations (Stewart, Field, & Echterling, 2016). What we experience in the world affects our behaviors, and our behaviors affect how we see the world. For example, many people will begin crying when they see someone else crying or even think of someone weeping; their mirror neurons are activated by the thought or sight of a person crying. They immediately feel an internal sensation of sadness, inducing them to cry even though they may not have felt sad a few moments before. These mirror neurons prompt children to imitate behaviors and emotional expressions. For example, when a child spontaneously begins to clap his hands in response to a strong rhythmic pulse, this action can also induce a more pleasant mood state and help "to regulate moods and emotions" (Trost, Labbé, & Grandjean, 2017, p. 96).

Entrainment shows how a child exposed to negative and traumatic relationships can unconsciously reenact this negativity, leading him to entrenched behaviors. Wholesome interactions within the therapy relationship may, in turn, be internalized by the child and strengthen his ability to respond more positively in general. In music, the interplay between therapist and child is based upon making satisfying sounds and rhythms, and in order to do so they must work together. By working together, a more positive style of response and reaction is developed, forming new memory traces and setting a foundation for growth.

By entraining to each other, individuals enter a common space of understanding and interaction. Stern (1985) frames this as an intersubjective space, where two people share in each other's experience. Winnicott (1971) describes this as the creative space of play between two people that is essential to a child's learning how to function in the world. Music can be used to create such a space that integrates physiological sensations, social behaviors, and emotions in a unique and powerful way (Trost et al., 2017).

ATTUNEMENT

Attunement is the process by which a person not only becomes sensitized to someone else's physical or emotional state, but also shares in the experience. When attuned to each other, two people get on the same wavelength, so to speak. They understand the other's thoughts and motivations and feel the essence of the other's emotional state. Stern (1985) focused on this intersubjective state as it develops between a mother and child, and sees this ability to sense what another person is feeling and shift your perception in order to share the feeling as a building block to emotional development. Parent and child communicate through sounds and actions that enliven the feelings both have. Attuning to each other is essential for a healthy relationship to develop and for the infant to feel loved and nurtured. An experience of mutual attunement "may lead to a feeling of being recognized on a nonverbal level and promote connectedness and coherence" (Trondalen & Skarderud, 2007, p. 106).

Attunement can also be understood to be the ability to sense what another person is feeling and adjust to meet that feeling. Heidegger (1995) writes, "It seems as though attunement is in each case already there, so to speak, like an atmosphere in which we first immerse ourselves and which then attunes us through and through" (pp. 66–67). His term "atmosphere" is apt in describing the somewhat ineffable process of attunement; it references a metaphysical perspective of how two human beings meet, sense each other's intentions and sensibilities, and interact. According to Heidegger, our relationships are predetermined by the climate in which we encounter each other and are influenced by nonverbal and noncognitive processes, notions that are supported by contemporary researchers and clinicians (Corbeil, Trehub, & Peretz, 2016; Tronick, 2007).

As a therapeutic principle, attunement is the bonding of therapist and child through child-directed work (Stewart et al., 2016). Therapists can also facilitate the attunement of parents/caregivers and their infants when dealing with attachment problems by focusing on mirroring and bodily sensations. This synchronization helps children "develop a sense of others' emotional states, which is a precursor of empathy" (Hart, 2017, p. 67). It moves beyond entrainment, for it is an ongoing process that, with careful thought and action, the therapist can focus on and develop to help a client feel safe. By absorbing and feeling some of what a client is experiencing, a therapist aligns herself with the client and creates a bridge of empathy and rapport. Kossak (2009) views attunement as an integral part of the therapeutic process, as it helps clients develop and sustain levels of intimacy. According to Kossak, "there is a direct correlation between experiencing intimacy and individual development, because it necessitates adaptations to changing needs, anxieties, and stresses that occur in relationships" (p. 15).

How to Attune to a Child through Music

Attunement is not only a psychological construct but also a potent musical process (Porges, 2009). Human communication is essentially musical in nature: we speak in phrases, emphasize rhythmic patterns, and use inflection (tonal movements upward or downward) to impart meaning and emotional vitality (Stern, 1985, 2010; Trevarthen, 1994). Acoustic analyses of parent–infant vocal interactions that occur when caregivers attune to their infants uncover an inborn musicality. The infant reveals his internal state in the musical elements of timing, intensity, and shape of his vocal sounds (Trondalen & Skarderud, 2007). The infant and parent instinctively regulate the pitch contours and inflections of each other's vocalizations (Trevarthen & Malloch, 2000). Humans have a strong, innate impulse to share feelings, and music is an expression of the quality of feeling that is being shared.

According to Trevarthen and Malloch (2000):

> Actually or potentially, making music is an act of intersubjectivity, a form of behavior that offers direct information on human motives, from which other humans can sense what underlies a person's actions and experience . . . this is because all humans act and may sympathize with movements of both body and voice that are rhythmic and melodic, with gestures linked into narrative cycles of expression. (p. 4)

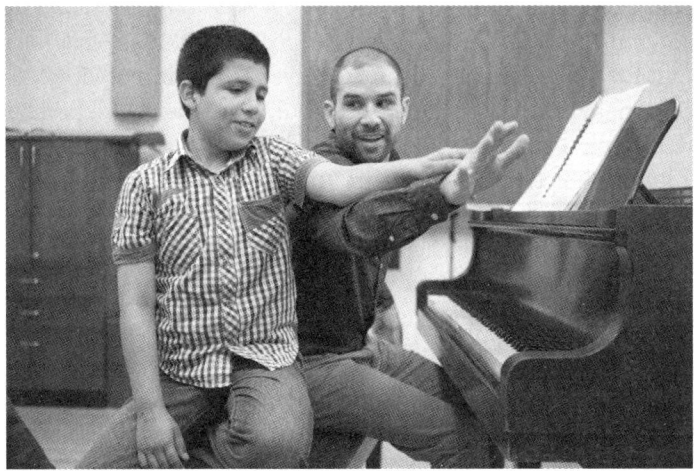

Boy singing at piano

The myriad methods a therapist uses to attune to her client can be thought of in musical terms. She can match the rhythm of speech: Is it fast or pressured or slow? Is the child's voice modulated or monotone? Does the therapist need to increase her speed/tempo in movements to match the child's energy? Is the child's tone of voice high- or low-pitched? What quality does the voice have: is it thin or reedy, or is its tone lower and body-centered? Does the therapist want to mirror movements and vocal quality, or provide a counterpoint, a different way to talk or move with the aim of helping the client self-regulate? Is the child rigid and fixed in how he talks and moves, or is he able to respond creatively and improvisationally to interactions? By thinking musically, it becomes easier for a therapist who works with children to bring music into the therapy room.

It is possible to use music to attune to children who may be unable to verbalize what may be overwhelming emotion. For example, when working with a very distressed 2-year-old boy with autism spectrum disorder, I (L. E. B.) began to vocalize, holding tones in a strong voice and adding rhythmic phrases to match his hiccupping crying sounds. After a minute or so he lifted his gaze to my face and began to stare intently at my mouth, as if in disbelief that I was making that sound. I continued to hold the tones but made them gentler and added a few lyrical motifs, all the while watching him as his face relaxed and his voice became softer. Suddenly we were singing together, making music with our voices. He lifted his hand and felt my mouth, throat, and jaw as I continued to create melodies that he responded to. His breathing became more regular and I started to sing the "The ABC Song" softly and slowly. The child became completely still and sighed deeply. I opened my bag of instruments and took out a hand drum. I played a few beats with my hands and then offered it to him. He reached out, took the drum, and began to explore it while I sang to him. When it came time to leave, his mother let me know that that was the first time she had seen him respond to someone else with such quiet attention.

In psychotherapy, the therapist is the instrument in that she makes changes in her posture, tone of voice, complexity of language, and facial expressions that create a presence of acceptance and build a bridge of empathy (Gil, 2015). By openly accepting the client as he presents himself, the therapist meets the client as he is. Making shifts in her demeanor and language in order to continually match, or attune to, the client's energetic and emotional manifestations builds the therapeutic relationship.

WORKING WITH CHILDREN WITH ATTACHMENT PROBLEMS

Winnicott's (1971) theory of the transitional object posits that the space between the client and the therapist is where trust is developed, where internal and external realities merge, and where therapeutic attachments are formed. When music is introduced into this space, a child is relieved of the pressure to verbalize by being given an alternate means of expressing his emotions. Further, music is a naturally integrative force. By virtue of its neurological and aesthetic effects, music can help develop the sense of self at the same time as building the therapeutic relationship.

Music holds the potential to transform a child's experience of himself even with the conscious use of a single tone. By taking a deep breath and vocalizing, a child emits a pure sound that has power and makes an aural impression on the immediate environment. To the child, this can feel cathartic: sustaining a note can be gratifying, calming, challenging, and fun. When supported or witnessed by the therapist, this act becomes interactive and empowering. In our work, we have seen many children who are initially unable to make contact through music in more than a fleeting manner. As they become more musically involved, they become capable of vocalizing one tone for longer periods of time. This note is symbolic of holding a relationship with themselves and with the music. When returned to in successive sessions, it is almost always accompanied by an increased strength in personality, expression, eye contact, and general presence.

Incorporating music into therapeutic interactions with children helps a therapist enter into the child's emotional world. When a child beats a drum vigorously, for example, it may sound like an expression of anger to a therapist who passively listens. However, when the therapist picks up another drum and beats in the same manner as the child, the sound can take on more meaning: it becomes energetic and expressive in its own right. It becomes an interactive activity that shifts the tenor of the play from angry to purposeful communication. Engaging in mutual musical expression can quickly transform an isolated emotional expression to a shared experience.

When a child is making music, it is important to observe *how* the child is playing: What are the qualities of the music? What is his energy level? Are his facial expressions congruent with how he is playing? Asking these questions can help a therapist quickly attune to the child's internal state and decide how to join in. You may choose to mirror the expressions and movements the child displays when playing. This is a supportive role that affirms that what the child is doing has meaning and prompts interaction. Or, you may choose to play differently from the child to offer an alternative form of expression. For example, playing in a manner that is opposite of how the child plays is another form of attunement that acts as a counterpoint to the child's expression. This can be an important intervention when you sense that the music the child plays has an undertone that is not healthy or productive.

By gently challenging the way a child plays, the therapist is symbolically, through sound, challenging the resistance (see Chapter 3) the child may be presenting in other areas of his life. For example, when a child who is being treated for attachment disorder first comes into the therapy room and immediately begins to beat a small hand drum and loudly sing a favorite song, he may reject the therapist's attempt to join in by playing or singing louder or shouting "No!" This may be indicative of the child's response to stressful or new situations—the child has a need to control the environment and self-soothe by singing a familiar song. Our recommendation here is for the therapist to mirror the child's body movements and affect, thereby underscoring the rhythmic nature of the child's music and offering a means of support. Holding steady in interacting with the child while respecting his boundaries might facilitate a more open interaction later on.

VIGNETTE

Fiona was adopted from Romania at age 16 months by an American family. Her early life in Romania had been spent first in an orphanage and then in an inadequate foster home where she had sometimes been tied to her crib. When she came to the United States, Fiona had some developmental delays and suffered from fears of abandonment, night terrors, and other significant attachment-related problems. She had a difficult adjustment to her new home life: she became emotionally withdrawn and developed autistic-like behaviors. She lost the language she had in the transition from Romanian to English, her play became disorganized and repetitive, and she clung to her adoptive mother. At just 16 months, she had suffered some major losses—that of her birth mother and her foster mother, as well as her familiar environment.

When I (J. C. B.) began seeing her for therapeutic music sessions, Fiona was 4 years old and had begun to develop a relationship with her adoptive mother. She was lively and outgoing and had done a significant amount of healing. Yet, she carried with her the trauma of her early life with its disrupted attachments. This manifested in low frustration tolerance, frequent and intense temper tantrums, perfectionism, and more. The mother, who was not musically inclined, recognized that Fiona loved music and was hoping that I could use music therapeutically to help her daughter cope with attachment issues and alleviate her troubling symptoms.

Fiona clearly felt at home in a musical environment; she loved to sing and play the various instruments. She brought in bags of stuffed animals from home each week and told stories, almost always related to the theme of exclusion—one animal was singled out for being different and was cruelly rejected and abused by the others. She would enact the same stories again and again, assigning roles to herself and to me, and telling me exactly what she wanted me to say. As is often true with children who have suffered trauma and negative early bonding experiences, she had a strong need to control the situation, including the music. I interpreted the exclusion theme in her play as an expression of her feeling like an outsider and not belonging anywhere. She was trying to find her own identity and her place in her family and in the world.

Whenever Fiona had an idea she wanted to express, she would spontaneously burst into song. It was through her singing that she could connect with her deepest emotions, singing about being overlooked and feeling all alone, wondering where she fit in, searching for a "real" family. She sang about wanting to cry, though she didn't know why, and of her yearning for someone to care for her. I supported her by singing with her, sometimes repeating her words and sometimes adding phrases to extend her ideas. I chose words that I imagined she was feeling. For example, one day she sang the words "I'm just all alone." I sang the phrase back to her, and she sang "With no one beside me." By connecting to my own feelings of sadness I was able to attune to her feelings of sadness in this shared intersubjective experience. I believe that she felt understood and less isolated since, in this song, she was not alone. The song unfolded like this:

> FIONA: I'm just all alone . . .
> THERAPIST: I'm just all alone . . .
> FIONA: With no one beside me . . .
> THERAPIST: No one to play with . . .
> FIONA: Or have fun with . . .

THERAPIST: I feel like I want to cry . . .

FIONA: Oohhh, I'm all alone.

Many times, she did not want any musical accompaniment; rather, she needed me to be a witness, someone who listened to her and allowed her voice to be heard, both literally and figuratively. Sometimes she incorporated the instruments in the room into her songs, and other times she did not. Having the instruments available, and knowing that I would support her musical efforts, gave her the freedom to be creative and express herself in a way that was satisfying to her. Within the safety of our relationship, and with me as her witness, partner, and empathetic reflection, she was able to gain a better sense of who she was and what kind of person she wanted to be. Singing about her innermost thoughts, emotions and conflicts allowed her to integrate the different aspects of herself that she was discovering. Our relationship and the attachment she formed with me helped to better equip her to form future attachments with others. For children like Fiona who naturally gravitate toward musical expression, offering this as a possibility can be tremendously important in their therapeutic process (Birnbaum, 2013).

VIGNETTE

Avala had been severely neglected by her parents who were methamphetamine addicts, and she was put into foster care at the age 2. At age 4, Avala starting meeting with Karl, a social worker who specialized in the treatment of abused and neglected children, for a series of play sessions. Avala was physically healthy but unable to make eye contact for more than a few seconds and resistant to any physical or emotional closeness. Her expressive language skills were assessed to be at the level of a 3-year-old child. She could form short, four- to five-word sentences yet struggled to speak complete sentences. She tended to answer questions with yes or no responses, without any further detail.

Avala was quickly drawn to the sand tray in Karl's office and spent her time arranging scenes, complete with figures and objects, and erasing them when she felt Karl's attention focused on her. Over the course of several sessions she began to relax in his presence and would tolerate him sitting next to her and watching her play. If he commented on her play, however, she shouted "No!" and pushed the sand to one side of the tray.

In their fourth session, Karl noted that Avala came into the therapy room with a smile on her face, as if she were looking forward to playing. He felt she was ready for more contact. When Avala began to play with the figures in the sand tray, Karl sat on the other side of the table and, without looking at her, began to vocalize rhythms and short melodies that matched how she placed the figures, how quickly she moved her hands, and the emotional quality of how they looked in the tray. When he started, Avala looked up at him but saw he was not looking at her, and she drew her gaze back to the sand tray and continued playing. Her movements began to slow down and become even more deliberate.

Karl continued vocalizing staccato phrases as well as longer melodies that arced either up or down, following the path of her movements. After a few minutes, Avala picked up one figure, that of a little girl, and waved it in the air as if the girl were flying. Karl matched this play with his voice, and Avala giggled. She then began to vocalize along with him, saying "whee" as she made the little girl swoop up and down. Their sounds blended to create an aural support for flying. Karl realized that he and Avala had attuned to each other. Their sounds entrained not only with each other but also with Avala's movements, reinforcing the vibrant musical connection they experienced. They both laughed at the same time, and Avala set the girl figure down gently onto the sand in a standing posture. After a few moments, Karl picked up another figure, this time a man, and vocalized "Hummm," as if wondering what to do with him. Avala looked up at him, her face rapt with attention, curious what would happen next. Karl knew this was a delicate moment. To him, in that moment the man figure represented all the men in Avala's short life. He set the man on the sand and began walking him around, vocalizing a light, happy tune using the sounds "tum-te-dum, tum-te-dum, daaa-da-da-da-daaa." He repeated the phrase several times and Avala joined in, singing the phrase with him. She picked up the girl figure and began walking her around the tray at the same time. The man and girl figures did not walk next to each other, but the parallel play and singing created an unseen bond between Karl and Avala, bringing them into a shared space of happy exploration and expression. After this interaction Avala turned away from the sand tray and spent the rest of the session coloring in a book, while Karl colored in a different book, next to her.

In their next session, they did not speak many words but engaged again in vocalizing to match their play. This time, Avala created a circle in the sand tray and in it placed a woman, man, and baby. Her vocalizing became flat, without any leaps or rhythms. Karl decreased the volume of his sounds so hers were most prominent. She moved the figures around in the circle, and then picked up the baby figure, cradling it in her hands. Karl vocalized a soft, long tone, and held it until his breath ran out. He then started the tone again, this time raising the pitch and volume a bit. Avala joined him in sounding this tone and together they held it as long as they could. It quickly transformed into a game, seeing who could hold the tone longer. Both of them started laughing, which made it impossible to hold the tone, which made them laugh harder. Avala and Karl looked at each other and next held the tone for as long as they could, then immediately started holding it again. They did this five times before becoming breathless, and while laughing Karl said, "Phew!," and Avala responded with, "That was fun! But I think I won!!" Lightheartedly, Karl said, "Well, I think I did pretty well, but yes, I do think you won that one!"

In thinking back on this session, Karl realized that Avala had not just sustained contact with him for almost 5 minutes; she had opened herself up to share a joyful experience with another person. She had willingly, and literally, held the interaction for a prolonged period, indicating that she was ready to engage with people around her. He was startled to realize that what he and Avala experienced in this session was what Maslow (1964) calls a peak experience: a shared time or intense engagement that had a timeless quality to it. This can also be thought of as a combination of emotional time and creative or now time, as described in Chapter 1. The connection they had made in their vocalizing together seemed to transcend words and everyday experiences. To Karl, it felt as if Avala had opened up parts of herself she had worked hard to keep hidden, and that she did so willingly and, perhaps, eagerly. He did not know what would come next but felt hopeful that Avala would continue to build on her ability to connect and express her feelings.

Karl took a chance when he used his voice in a new way. This approach may seem intimidating to some therapists, yet we encourage you to tap into the part of you that once used your voice freely and openly. Becoming child-like in this instance means going back to a time when you felt it was okay to sing silly songs, make rhythmic noises, and let your voice be the signal to others of how you were feeling. In the "Recommendations for Practice" at the end of this chapter we offer some tips on how to reconnect with your voice in a conscious manner, with the intention of becoming freer with it in therapeutic situations.

WORKING WITH PARENTS AND CAREGIVERS

Working with music is a powerful intervention, as the interplay of vocalizations, sounds, and movement that occurs between parent and child is the foundation of communication and is also a musical relationship (Trevarthen & Malloch, 2000). For example, a mother intuitively raises and lowers the pitch of her voice when cooing to her baby; rocking her baby to sleep is a natural way of using rhythmic movement to soothe him. Trevarthen and Malloch (2000) also note a parallel between the parent–infant dyad and the therapist–client dyad. The therapeutic relationship between therapist and client is in some respects a reenactment of the parent–child bond, and as such can serve as the mechanism for change and growth.

Developmental psychologists such as Stern (1985, 2010) and Trevarthen (1994) have found that babies are born fully equipped and motivated to participate in reciprocal communication with others. Mothers and babies can "read" and respond to each other's signals, which serves as the foundation for emotional attunement. Both mother and baby exercise some control in responding to and eliciting responses from the other through playful sounds, short (three- to four-note) melodies, babbling, and cooing.

There has been a great deal of research on effective attachment-based interventions with at-risk families (Berlin, Ziv, Amaya-Jackson, & Greenberg, 2007; Stewart et al., 2016). These include video-based programs that enable caregivers to observe their own moment-by-moment interactions with their infants or toddlers. The COS intervention (Powell et al., 2014), described earlier, provides parents with the tools to be nurturing and protective while supporting the child's exploration and independence. Attunement to the baby's signals and cues and providing a resonant response are significant elements of this approach.

Music is also powerful when working with parents of older children because it can serve as an equalizer and mediator when there are difficulties or issues in parent–child relationships. When two people are playing music, they can take turns determining how the music should sound. Giving power to the child to lead—for example, by deciding what dynamic his parent should play on hand drums—equalizes the inherent power dynamic that exists in parent–child interactions. This can be important for both the child and the parent: the child feels like he is being heard and has some control, while the parent has to listen and respond to the child's wishes. This can lead to new insights for a parent:

the child may have valuable ideas to contribute or may present himself with a level of confidence the parent had not noticed before. Engaging in music and vocal play also helps the parent attune to the child's proclivity to respond to music and interact in a way that precludes the need for verbal language skills (Zeifman & Hazan, 2016).

VIGNETTE

Even a sensitive parent who is generally attuned to her child can misread her child's cues. I (J. C. B.) began seeing Luke, a boy with global developmental delays due to a genetic disorder, when he had just turned 2 years old. He was not yet walking or talking but was alert and aware of his surroundings. He seemed to be an easygoing and happy child who had healthy attachments; his parents and 4-year-old sister doted on him. Luke was reaching developmental milestones, albeit slowly. His mother, Carrie, was willing to do all she could to give her son opportunities to develop his skills and asked to be part of the therapy sessions. He was already receiving speech and occupational therapy in a home-based early intervention program. She knew that he loved music—whenever he heard music being played he would stop whatever he was doing and respond by smiling, bouncing, and clapping his hands. Carrie was eager for him to develop language, and this was what prompted her to take him to a form of therapy that incorporated music. When treatment began, he made very few vocal sounds and had no words; he was learning a few signs to help him communicate.

I played guitar and sang while sitting close to Luke so that he could easily see the movements of my mouth—this seemed to fascinate him and he stared intently at my face. He also was drawn to the sound of the guitar, reaching out to strum the strings. One of my initial goals was that he become comfortable exploring his own voice, as a precursor to speech. In the early sessions he was quiet, though he seemed to be taking it all in: the new room, new person with an unfamiliar voice, and the sounds of the various instruments he was given to explore. To encourage him to vocalize, I introduced animal puppets and made up a song about the different sounds they made. I invited Carrie to join in the singing, which she was happy to do. Luke was interested in the puppets, touching their eyes, ears, nose, and tail, and I sang about these body parts. Still, he did not try making any sounds himself.

One day a few weeks later, while we were singing the animal song that was now familiar to him, Luke opened his mouth wide and made a short *ah* sound. I repeated his sound, singing it in the pitches of the melody so that it became part of the song. Hearing his sound reflected back to him encouraged him to continue vocalizing, and the three of us—me, Luke, and Carrie—engaged in a playful musical exchange using the syllable "ah." Luke began to sustain his sound ("*aaahhhhh*") and smiled with delight. Carrie was also delighted with this new development, seeing a door open to her son's acquisition of speech, and told me that she wanted him to try more sounds, using other vowels and consonants. As she quickly began to introduce new sounds, her face became quite serious and her body tense. Luke seemed to sense his mother's anxiety and feel her pressure, and he stopped responding. The smile faded from his face and he took on a worried expression.

I explained to Carrie that Luke needed a chance to enjoy and master his new ability to say *ah* and that he might not yet be ready to try a range of sounds. Her anxiety about Luke's language delay interfered with her ability to read her son's cues and attune to his needs. Caregivers and therapists can support and provide opportunities for development to unfold, but we cannot force it. I encouraged Carrie to relax and to be playful in the vocal exchanges, and not to push Luke—it was important that the vocal play be fun for them both. When she was able to put her concerns aside, focus on the interaction in the moment, and take her cues from Luke, he once again began to joyfully explore vocally and embraced his mother's participation.

Lessons from a Neonatal Intensive Care Unit

Parents of infants in a neonatal intensive care unit (NICU) often experience high levels of anxiety and are apprehensive about their child's prognosis and development (Bieleninik, Ghetti, & Gold, 2016; Schlez et al., 2011). Their ability to bond with their baby is severely hampered by the environment, fear of harming an already fragile child, constant medical interventions, and simply not knowing how to be engaged in the healing process. Parents can misinterpret their child's vocalizations, especially when in a pressured environment like the NICU. A high, thin cry with an accompanying fist in the air can be mistaken for a cry of hunger when it may be more indicative of the infant being overstimulated (Loewy, 2007). Helping parents differentiate between cries and practice responding to fussy cries with low, soothing melodies or vocalizations can make them feel more confident and in tune with their child's needs. Providing family-centered and culturally sensitive therapy is important as parents will need these skills when they return home with their infants.

Encouraging parents to find meaningful songs and listening alongside them creates a shared space. This may be a time for a therapist, nurse, or child life specialist to set aside their own musical preferences, for inevitably the music a child has listened to in the womb and the parents' preferences are the best sources for songs that may be useful therapeutically. For example, one mother who was visiting her baby in the NICU said she listened to a lot of music by the band Nirvana when she was pregnant. When one of the Nirvana songs was played live by a musician in a slower tempo and at a low volume (see below), the child's heartrate and respiration rate immediately decreased, showing a shift into a more relaxed state. According to Porges, "sucking, swallowing, vocalizations, heart rate, and bronchial constriction are regulated by a common brainstem area" (2011, p. 90). Singing with a low, soothing tone does more than evoke a relaxation response; it gives the infant a healthy stimulus that has far-ranging physiological benefits.

Please note that we do not advocate that therapists use live or loud music in the NICU setting because there are specific, medically necessary boundaries regarding the types of music a baby born prematurely can withstand. Even when parents choose music that is not suitable for playing in the NICU area, these songs may still be a resource for a therapist: listening to the songs away from the unit or talking about the lyrics with the parents may lead to discussions that might otherwise be difficult. Finding songs that are meaningful to parents allows them to begin processing their emotions. Loewy (2015) refers to what she calls "songs of kin," or family-preferred songs, that reflect culture and heritage. These help parents and family members bring their full sense of identity into the session and helps them cope with the stresses they encounter. Honoring the culture parents come from is an essential element of comprehensive and holistic care (Mondonaro, 2016).

VIGNETTE

Mariana was a child psychologist working on a NICU. One day, she noticed a father, grandmother, and two small children in the private waiting room. She knew the mother was still on the maternity ward and that the baby boy, born 6 weeks prematurely, had been having difficulty breathing on his own. She also knew that the family spoke Spanish and little English. When she went to greet them, she noticed the father looked exhausted, and grandmother anxious. The children, ages 3 and 5, were running around the room playing tag. Mariana had a Bluetooth speaker connected to her phone and brought up "Buenas Noches," or as English-speaking people know it, "Are You Sleeping?" As soon as the music began playing the children came over to her to listen, then began to sing along. Father and grandmother watched, smiling, and looked energized. Mariana spoke Spanish and was able to ask the children what other songs they like, or what songs their mother liked. The older child immediately said "La Bicicleta!" Mariana found this song on her phone and played it. The children and grandmother clapped along enthusiastically. When it finished Mariana commented on the love and happiness expressed in the room. This led to a lively discussion of how the children hoped the baby could come home soon and how much they loved him. Both the grandmother and father nodded their heads in agreement and shared some of their worries and fears. The music presented an opportunity for these family members to come together, relax for a few minutes, and unite in their love and hope.

Music can help parents and family members tap into their strengths, connect with memories, and better understand the many changes they are going through. I (L. E. B.) was leaving the NICU one day and decided to check in on a mother I had seen earlier. Her parents were with her, and her grandmother was holding the baby. I asked if they would like to hear one more song and, when they agreed, I instinctively chose "Isn't She Lovely" by Stevie Wonder. I sang it in a much slower tempo and in a waltz rhythm, and the mother sang along. When I finished the song, the mother teared up and said her husband had sung that song to her during her pregnancy when she was feeling "particularly unlovely." We talked as a group about some of the changes the entire family had faced, and how they needed to support each other. The song led to a meaningful exploration of their feelings and fears surrounding the premature birth of the baby.

VIGNETTE

Hospital psychologist Courtney walked through the NICU and noticed one mother, Jang-mi, sitting by her baby's bed with her hands in her lap and a nervous expression on her face. Courtney approached Jang-mi and asked her how she was doing, to which Jang-mi replied, "I am okay, thank you." Her child, Hyuk, had been born 4 weeks early with respiratory issues. Courtney offered to meet with Jang-mi to talk about how she was feeling, and Jang-mi said "Yes, that would be wonderful." They agreed to meet later that day in Courtney's office.

During their session, Jang-mi shared her anxiety over Hyuk's fragile physical state and her frustration that she could do little more than pump breast milk for him. Courtney asked her how she felt when she held Hyuk, and Jang-mi said, "Happy but so nervous!" With that information, Courtney was able to talk with Jang-mi about the importance of breathing deeply and audibly when she was near Hyuk, and how this type of breathing has physical and emotional benefits for not only Hyuk, but also for her. Together they practiced taking deep breaths, making the exhales audible. After a few breaths, Jang-mi said, "I feel so much more relaxed. You are saying Hyuk will also feel relaxed if I do this?" Courtney shared that research has shown that breathing this way is something that babies attune to; they automatically respond by breathing more deeply themselves (Loewy et al., 2013). It also helps them tune out the sounds of the NICU.

Courtney then asked if Jang-mi ever sang lullabies to Hyuk and Jang-mi responded that she had been singing, but very softly so as not to disturb anyone around her. She said she had several favorite Korean lullabies that her own mother had sung to her. Courtney shared that lullabies are good medicine for babies in the NICU, with their steady tempo, predictable structure, and limited number of notes. They talked a little about the importance of these elements, and suddenly Jang-mi exclaimed, "So it is good to sing lullabies to him?" Courtney assured her it was and said it might also make her feel less helpless and closer to him. Jang-mi said, "I am going back right now to sing to him!" and thanked Courtney for her time. Together they walked back to the NICU, and Courtney stood just outside the room and watched as Jang-mi pulled her chair up close to Hyuk's crib, leaned her head in close to his, and began to sing softly. She then reached out and began to stroke his head gently as she sang.

When Courtney saw Jang-mi next, she asked how everything was going. Jang-mi expressed her gratitude, saying, "When I went in and began to sing to him, he was fussy and crying a little. Within a couple of minutes, he stopped fussing. I remembered the importance of exhaling so he could hear me and began to do this, and he opened his eyes, looked up at me, and sighed a little! I was so happy! I have had some very loving moments with him."

WORKING WITH GROUPS AND PEER RELATIONSHIPS

Music can be a solitary experience as listening to music, singing, or playing an instrument are often pursuits done alone. Remembering or thinking about a piece of music, a process called audiation, is also a solo experience, albeit satisfying. Yet music can be used as effectively for promoting group attunement and social interaction (Davies, Barwick, & Richards, 2015). As shown earlier, music can easily be shared between two people by singing, playing, or listening together, or by one person performing while the other listens and bears witness. It can also be an engaging and powerful group experience, bringing people together for a common, positive purpose. Working with others toward achieving a mutual goal fosters a sense of belonging and community. When children attune to others' needs they learn tolerance and respect for individual differences. In the group setting, children feel pride in sharing their own accomplishments while delighting in the achievements of other group members. Children who have difficult interpersonal relationships can learn prosocial behaviors such as turn taking, empathy, and listening through group experiences (Eisenberg, Spinrad, & Valiente, 2017; Brief & Motowidlo, 1986). According to Knight, Spiro, and Cross (2017), collective musical behaviors "afford the perception of actions, intentions

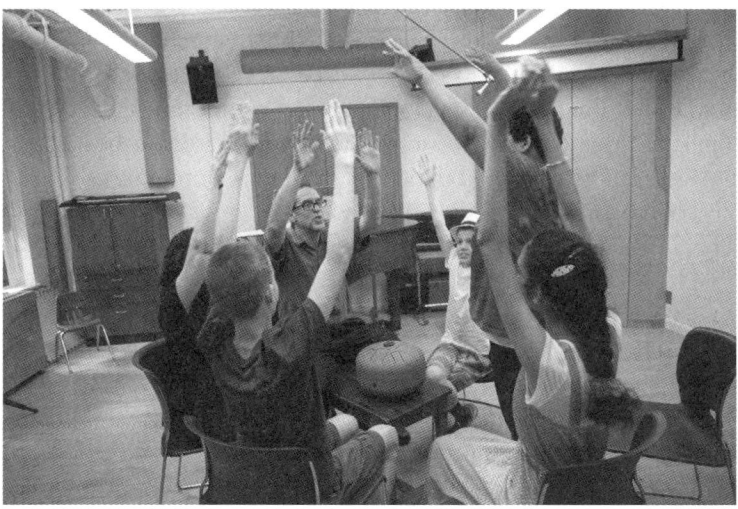

Group of children

and motivational states as *joint* action, *shared* intentionality and *mutual* motivational states, which in turn fosters interpersonal affiliation and prosocial behaviours, including trust" (p. 99).

Music can also be used to facilitate discussion and interpersonal work as group members share their thoughts and ideas and give honest yet caring feedback to others. When we listen, play music, or sing in a group, we become more aware of other people and develop a sense of belonging to something larger than oneself. This phenomenon is seen throughout society: singing the national anthem before a ballgame unifies the crowd; singing in places of worship promotes a feeling of spiritual connection among members. Music plays a part in many life rituals—weddings and funerals, for example—that deepen a shared emotional experience. Children with emotional and developmental challenges may have limited means to achieve this sense of community that is such a vital part of psychological health, and music can provide an avenue for doing so. Musical interactions lend themselves easily to turn taking, whether it be singing phrases back and forth or taking turns tapping rhythmic phrases on a drum. This back-and-forth exchange is the foundation of human conversation. Children may find it easier to access this kind of mutual interaction through music than through verbal means.

I (J. C. B.) was working in a school for children with language-based learning disabilities doing group music activities. One such activity was an enactment of a story based on the Grimm fairy tale "Fair Katrinelje and Pif-Paf-Poltrie." Nordoff and Robbins (1961) have written music and text to turn the story into a "musical working game for children." One day, it was 9-year-old Melvin's turn to take on the role of Pif. Melvin was what you might call the class clown, always trying to get his classmates to laugh. He was regularly sent to the principal's office because of his disruptive behavior. We had done this story many times in the class, and the children were very familiar with the songs and knew what was going to happen. At the end of the story, Pif is required to sweep up the leaves that had been scattered all over the room. The psychological impact of the story concerns cleaning up one's mess, both literally and symbolically. The music that accompanies Pif's sweeping is solemn yet supportive, underscoring the seriousness of the task Pif has undertaken. As Melvin swept the leaves into a pile in the center of the room, the other children listened to the music and watched silently, in rapt attention. Melvin worked carefully to successfully accomplish his difficult task. When he had finished, there was a smile and a glowing look of pride on his face. After that day, there was a noticeable change in both Melvin and his classmates. They seemed to see him differently, not merely as a goofy kid but as someone they could take seriously—he had earned their respect. And Melvin himself had changed—he now could see himself not only as someone who needed to act up to gain the attention and admiration of his peers, but as someone who was competent and able to accomplish positive things. By immersing himself in the task of "sweeping up the mess" with the support of his classmates and together with the aural soundscape of solemn intention, he was able to move beyond his clownish identity and establish himself as a caring and responsible peer. While it is possible that the story could be told without music, the music adds emotional depth and pulls the children in so that they care about the idiosyncratic characters in this old and quaint tale.

SUMMARY

In this chapter, we discuss the many ways music fits into theories of attachment, including biobehavioral models like polyvagal theory and attachment interventions like the COS. By making and listening to music, we naturally engage in processes of entrainment and attunement; these terms even have musical roots and meanings. When working with attachment issues, music offers clinicians a means to connect with, support, and encourage new insights and ways for parents to be with their children. Theorists are finding new links between dysfunctional attachments and responses to trauma (Ogden & Fisher, 2015); having a foundational knowledge of the role music can play in the treatment of children with attachment difficulties helps us move next into the discussion of how music can play a part in psychotherapy with children who have trauma-related issues.

RECOMMENDATIONS FOR PRACTICE

- Practice vocalizing, becoming more confident in your use of your voice. Making up short songs to the beat of the windshield wipers frees your imagination and prompts you to sing in a spontaneous way. Many of the children seen in psychotherapy have not had typical childhoods and were deprived of some of the joyful aspects of this time in their lives. Being willing to come up with rhythms, phrases, and melodies that fit the moment allows a child to reconnect with his own sense of spontaneity. Karl spent time singing long tones in preparation for some of his work with Avala. Make a game of holding a note like Karl did.

- If you are not comfortable using your voice, role playing with a vocal coach is a way to develop confidence. You can experiment with being the child or therapist.
- Play an "emotions game." Becoming more regulated in emotional expression requires a child to be able to identify different emotions. Making a game of identifying an emotion can be fun and satisfying, while offering the child an opportunity to feel more in control.
  - Start simply, with two hand drums. Give brief instructions like "Let's see if you can tell what emotion I am playing" and then play a short pattern that indicates a happy, angry, or sad mood. A happy mood might have a light, skipping feeling to it; an angry mood might be expressed by a loud, faster pattern; and a sad mood might be softer and slower.
  - Let the child take a turn playing the emotion and making you guess.
  - When you have gone through this practice several times, bring another instrument in that requires more control. For example, a larger drum that the child must balance on his legs, or a metallophone that requires dexterity to get the sound just right.
- Make up songs. Listen to the sounds in the environment and make up short songs about what these sounds are. You can get a little silly with this game and pretend the sounds are something very different, for example, instead of singing about the rain falling on the roof, sing about little fingers drumming on the roof—who could be doing this?!
- Pay close attention to the rhythmic and melodic elements of the child's music. Listen for the music in the child's speech or play. Be aware of the difference between mirroring, or answering, and mimicking a child's sounds: mirroring can be experienced as a supportive gesture, a kind of conversation, while mimicking sounds exactly can feel intrusive.
- Reflect the tempos, rhythms, and pitches of the child's music and respond by making your own sounds that complement his.
- Match the child's energy level and then gradually introduce the opposite energy level until a balance is achieved.
- Introduce variation through tempo and/or dynamic changes, or through use of different instruments, and invite the child to vary and develop his ideas.

- Sing about what the child is doing—this validates the child and makes him feel important and understood. This can lead into a kind of game where your singing and the child's play then become a form of interaction that creates a positive relationship between you.
- Creating playlists with parents for their own relaxation and for listening with their baby fosters bonding and gives them something concrete and enjoyable to do. When meeting with parents for the first time, include music preferences in your initial interview questions. Ask if there are any specific songs that are special to parents, either singly or as a couple. Suggest that you help them create a playlist of songs to listen to that are particularly meaningful or helpful when dealing with any stresses they may be having with their newborn or infant.
- Work with parents on developing breathing techniques. Breathing in deeply to a slow count of 4, holding the breath with a count of 2, and breathing out with a count of 4 can stimulate a relaxation response. This is helpful for parents to practice for their own stress relief, and to become more comfortable modeling deep breathing with their infant.
- Using lullabies in the treatment setting can have an effect on children. Pretending to sleep or having dolls "sleep" to recorded songs with steady tempos and few notes (e.g., "Twinkle, Twinkle, Little Star" or "Are You Sleeping?") deepens the experience and encourages the child to relax.

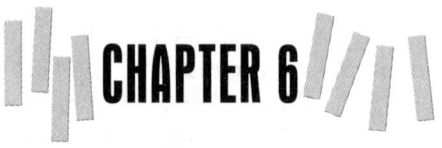

Trauma and Resilience

> Through improvisation, composing, listening, and various creative experiences with music, the survivor can connect with what he or she could not express verbally and begin to rebuild a new sense of normal in life.
> —BORCZON (2015, p. 399)

Trauma is widespread in our modern world; harrowing or painful events are at the root of many human difficulties. There are many possible sources of trauma, including inadequate or unhealthy family situations; emotional, physical, or sexual abuse; sudden loss; natural disasters; experiencing or witnessing violence or acts of war; bullying; accidents; serious illness or medical procedures, and more. What is traumatic for one child may be tolerated well by another, for responses to trauma are highly personal. Studies suggest that over half the general population has been exposed to major trauma, and up to 40% of traumatized children develop adverse psychiatric and psychological reactions to trauma (Saxe, Ellis, & Brown, 2015).

Children who have suffered some sort of abuse, neglect, or emotional or physical trauma cope with the effects and aftermath in ways that are unique to their family history, culture, developmental stage, and physiology. When children who have experienced trauma do not process their experience, they often show an increase in negative behaviors (Carey, 2006). They may become hyperactive or completely shut down. They may talk nonstop about everything except the trauma, or they may speak very little to anyone. When children experience a trauma, the brain responds by blocking emotional pathways. The child's affect may be flat, and he may have a limited range of emotional expression. The child is often psychologically exhausted and disinterested in engaging in social or therapeutic interactions (Malchiodi, 1998). The ability to self-regulate is compromised and there are implications for life-long issues with depression, poor social relations, and distorted emotional processing (Afolabi, 2015).

Much has been written about the mind–body connection in trauma, and how trauma symptoms remain in the body (Levine & Frederick, 1997; Scaer, 2014). It is as if the trauma is still happening days, weeks, or even years later. The child may not feel connected to his body nor grounded in the "here and now." He may be hypervigilant toward potential threats, both real and imagined. Perhaps the most salient characteristics of someone who has suffered trauma are a sense of helplessness and loss of control. The individual feels overwhelmed by his feelings but unable to do anything about them. This "freeze response" is a reaction to fear; a person may "shut down" or withdraw in an effort to protect himself (Scaer, 2014). Finding ways to bring music into the therapy room can help unlock memories and aid in processing traumatic events. Music can help to reshape the physiological response to trauma. The natural response to music is healthy and can be tapped into and focused on as a means of building resilience. Similar to art and play therapy approaches that "support resilience and enhance posttraumatic growth through sensory-based methods [and] capitalize on right-brain-dominant, action-oriented experiences" (Malchiodi, 2015, p. 129), strategies that rely upon music activate strengths and capabilities not accessible through words alone.

PROCESSING TRAUMA THROUGH MUSIC

A child who suffers from a trauma can have long-term issues "with affect dysregulation, aggressions against self and others, dissociative symptoms, somatization, and character pathology. These various symptoms tend to cluster into distinct patterns and to be highly interrelated" (van der Kolk, Roth, Pelcovitz, Sunday, & Spinazzola, 2005, pp. 395–396). There is a dissonance among thoughts, feelings, and actions, and the child experiences his internal world as chaotic and disorganized. One reason to bring music into the therapy room is that it is a naturally structured experience (Beer, 2011). Music, in the broadest sense, can be defined as organized sound (Varèse & Wen-Chung, 1966). The aural organization of music can bring a sense of internal stability and security to a child who is simply listening to a song. A well-chosen piece of music can override the disabling effects of trauma and help build mastery and self-control, two things essential to recovery (van der Kolk et al., 2005). Experiencing music, whether through playing or listening, with another person can be a nonthreatening way to work through altered relationships. It can be easier to trust someone when you do not always need to talk to them about highly charged issues.

There are many facets of helping children to process trauma through music. These include:

- Addressing the physiological response to trauma.
- Building safety and trust.
- Fostering strength, control, and resilience.
- Facilitating emotion regulation.
- Addressing the dissociative aspects of trauma.

Addressing the Physiological Response to Trauma

Trauma affects children not just emotionally and psychologically, but also physically—the body responds by becoming "hyperaroused" (Levine & Frederick, 1997; Lyon, D'Antonio, & Beck, 2014). Children may become exquisitely sensitive to any perceived danger and react accordingly. This neurological response to trauma is natural and happens consistently among children and adults. They are caught in a fight/flight/freeze dynamic that is confusing and chaotic. It has been well documented that the physiological response to trauma alters the biochemistry of the brain (Bromberg, 2006; Perry & Szalavitz, 2006). These changes may be adaptive for a child in a threatening or dangerous situation, but they are maladaptive if they continue once the child returns to normal conditions. The resulting posttraumatic stress disorder (PTSD) can interfere with typical development and learning, and lead to emotional and behavioral problems.

Children often have difficulty talking about their trauma (Levine & Frederick, 1997; Perry & Szalavitz, 2006). This is largely due to the fact that traumatic memories are stored in the limbic portion of the brain, which is primarily responsible for feelings and emotions, not language and reasoning. The memories are stored as emotions, body sensations, and sensory images such as sounds, smells, and visual images (van der Kolk et al., 2005).

Music has tremendous potential for helping children who have been traumatized and who are not able to access their memories through verbal means. Music can stabilize physiological responses, thereby increasing a client's ability to self-soothe and regulate (Hodges & Sebald, 2011).

This allows a child to begin to be able to remember and work through the event that activated the traumatic condition, and to regain a sense of emotional stability (Davis, 2010).

Although physiological responses are not limited to children who experience physical injuries, the following paragraphs focus on this population because approximately five children out of every 100 are hospitalized for a major medical emergency, illness, or accident. While "the majority of pediatric patients and their families are resilient and do well" (National Child Traumatic Stress Network [NCTSN], n.d.-b, p. 11), the potential to develop traumatic stress disorders and maladaptive psychological responses is ever-present. One in five children who suffer a major injury, and even their parents, will exhibit symptoms of PTSD up to 4 months after the accident (Winston, Kassam-Adams, Garcia-España, Ittenbach, & Cnaan, 2003). Frequently, child patients are not informed about why they are being treated, reinforcing feelings of helplessness and disempowerment (NCTSN, n.d.-b). If the stress of being hospitalized is not addressed, the after-effects of trauma can be long-lasting.

Many children respond to the stresses of being on a pediatric ward with fear, withdrawal from interactions, and anger. Resistance to undergoing invasive medical procedures takes various forms that can make it difficult for doctors and nurses to provide care; children become fearful and parents become protective. Psychologists and child life specialists work to normalize the hospital environment and tap into a child's existing ego strengths. These specialists use a variety of techniques to help calm children, yet often music is left out of their therapeutic toolbox due to uncertainty about how to use the modality (Beer & Lee, 2017). Bringing music into a session with a hospitalized or otherwise traumatized child can help the child reconnect with his preinjury or pretraumatized self. Talking about and listening to favorite pieces of music, rewriting lyrics to familiar songs, or singing together can alleviate worry and refocus the child on what is fun and familiar to him. The vignette below highlights issues relating to hospitalized children; these techniques are also useful for children who do not have physical injuries.

VIGNETTE

Mike was a young child who had been in a horrific car accident that seriously injured his father. The accident took place on a hot summer night, just a few months before his fourth birthday. His father had taken him to the playground while his mother stayed behind with his baby sister. On their way home, another driver sped through a stop sign, t-boning their car on the driver's side. As his father was being treated by paramedics, Mike was put in the ambulance and taken to the hospital. One of the paramedics said, "I felt so bad. The kid was clearly able to see his dad lying on the ground and was shouting 'Daddy!' over and over."

Two days later, Mike was still in the hospital being treated for a concussion while his father was in the intensive care unit in a medically induced coma. Previously a bubbly, quick-to-laugh boy, he spoke few words and made no eye contact with anyone other than his mother. He yelled out when doctors examined him, and when his mother Anne visited him he was anxious and continually asked about his father. The pediatric unit's social worker, Kailey, asked Anne to bring him familiar toys and books, yet nothing seemed to hold much interest for him. When Kailey attempted to engage him in therapeutic play or conversation about his interests, he turned away from her and closed his eyes. She also talked to him, explaining why he was in the hospital and how he would be able to go home soon, and spent time reading his favorite books with him. He engaged with her while looking at the books yet only glanced at her sideways, and rarely with a smile. Anne shared that he had always loved to sing and was always making up "funny little songs about whatever he was doing." Kailey had sung in her college choir and wondered if singing might be a way to help Mike open up.

The day after talking with Anne, Kailey went into Mike's room and greeted him. He looked up at her but did not respond verbally. After pulling a chair up close to his bed, she reached into her bag, retrieved two small hand drums and placed them on his bedside table, then took a couple of deep, audible breaths, sighing gently as she breathed out. She noticed that on the third breath Mike breathed in deeper and seemed to relax a bit after breathing out. As soon as this moment of relaxation occurred, a hospital cart wheeled by his room noisily, startling them both. Mike looked up at Kailey in surprise and they spontaneously smiled at each other. Kailey sang "Such a loud and noisy cart, noisy cart, noisy cart, such a loud and noisy cart, going by the room" to the tune of "Mary Had a Little Lamb." Her gaze was turned toward the door and away from him when she heard him laugh—a quick, short laugh, but a laugh nevertheless. He said, half-singing, "Noisy cart, noisy cart, don't go by my room." Kailey picked up on this and chanted, "When I want to sleep it's noisy cart, noisy cart, going by my room." Still without looking directly at him, she picked up one of the hand drums and then, looking over at him, offered it to him. He took the drum and began to play rhythmically in the speaking pattern of "noisy cart." She picked up the other drum and played a soft, steady beat to support his playing. When he stopped after a few rounds of "noisy cart," she kept the beat going and half-spoke and half-sang "There's so many things going on." Mike responded quietly, "Yes there are, so many things, I just want to go home!" Kailey continued the steady beat and half-sang, "What do you miss about home?" Their playing and chanting continued, with Mike expressing what he missed about home while rhythmically beating the drum in time with the syllables he spoke. After 10 minutes of playing and singing/talking, he seemed to tire, so Kailey asked if he wanted to stop for now and maybe play again later. He looked directly at her and nodded in agreement. She asked him if he might want to make up a song about going home and he replied "uh-huh."

Children spontaneously create songs, with content ranging from comments on their actual activity, to fanciful imagination, to made-up words and sounds. Singing is empowering (Austin, 2002)—the voice is a personal reflection of who we are. Singing together with another person can be an intimate human connection. Writing or improvising a song about the child's experience, like Kailey did with Mike, can provide a much-needed sense of power over the trauma.

In subsequent sessions, Kailey brought the hand drums to continue this familiar way of interacting with Mike. The drumming and chanting they first engaged in became a foundation for other interactions. Mike chose a song, "The Wheels on the Bus," to use to write a song about going home. The melody offered a safe and predictable form for him to express himself, and Kailey helped Mike write new lyrics. He also opened up verbally, asking her about his father and about the accident. He began to smile while they made up some silly lyrics, such as "the wheels on the cart are way too loud!" to the tune of "The Wheels on the Bus." It became a running joke between them, and whenever the cart went by the room they would both chant "noisy cart."

In reviewing her work with Mike, Kailey realized the rhythmic play helped him interact with her in a nonthreatening manner. His ability to engage in steady drumming while he played and chanted was crucial to helping him stabilize emotionally and feel safe. Their playing together was symbolic of his ability to interact in a meaningful and communicative way, yet he was also able to play separately on his own drum and thereby maintain a sense of independence. Kailey viewed the occurrence of the cart going by as symbolic of the lack of control Mike had over his environment, yet in naming it and singing about it he was able to master his response to it. Kailey recognized that by not verbalizing what could possibly be going on with him or how tough it was to be in the hospital, she had given him a chance to musically voice his reactions and regain a sense of his pre-accident personality. He was able, through this musical exchange, to begin to work through the trauma he had suffered.

Another aspect of this story that needs to be emphasized is that using this approach with children in a hospital setting, who are either getting ready to undergo a procedure or recovering from a trauma, has physical benefits. The act of singing opens the lungs and increases the flow of oxygen to the brain. Playing the drum activates motor neurons and releases endorphins. Singing and playing music rejuvenates the mind and body and creates new pathways of neural connection. In essence, music as a whole-brain phenomenon stimulates growth-oriented change and helps children experience connection to others and joy in music making.

Building Safety and Trust

Beyond physiological and neurological responses, children who have suffered trauma may experience greater amounts of stress and depression, and isolate themselves from others (Briere & Scott, 2014). They may keep their trauma a secret, and not sharing it may lead to feelings of deep loneliness. Allowing others to see their pain and to comfort them is a critical step in healing.

Finding ways to build, or rebuild, a child's sense of safety and trust is a prerequisite for all therapeutic relationships. It is common for children to experience a rupture in their sense of personal boundaries and become unable to differentiate healthy versus unhealthy boundaries (Afolabi, 2015). There are particular issues related to trust to consider when working with music. As shown in the above vignette about Mike, music can be a potent means of connecting with a child and establishing a sense of safety and trust. However, music's inherent power to evoke emotion can bring forth unexpected responses that may leave a client feeling out of control and a therapist uncertain what to do next. Mental health clinicians wanting to use music in their practice should be aware that music is processed differently than words and can bring up emotions directly related to the trauma that may be too intense or frightening during early stages of therapy. Music has the potential to quickly and immediately access sources of trauma or activate traumatic memories, and so a clinician needs to be especially aware of the need to create a slower pace or to pause a music experience at the first sign of a client becoming overwhelmed (Robarts, 2016). Indeed, the use of music in treating trauma calls for caution, but there are many simplified rhythmic and melodic strategies therapists can use in their work. A therapist can always stop the music and return to verbal processing of the material when emotions become too sharp or intensify unexpectedly. The following vignette illustrates some of these techniques and issues.

VIGNETTE

Kumala, a music therapy colleague, shared a story that provides insight into how to use music with traumatized children and teens. She was working at a residential youth facility where she conducted music therapy groups with clients in the 10- to 12-year age range. The social worker, Tony, had noticed how well the children in the group responded to music—they were talking, interacting, and working together. In particular, he noticed that Brad, a boy who had been molested the previous year by a family friend, was engaged during music therapy sessions. Brad refused to talk in his individual therapy sessions with Tony and was resistant to sand play, puppets, and other play therapy interventions.

One day Tony took Kumala aside and asked for her advice. He told her that he had tried to bring music into his sessions with Brad and had contacted Brad's mother to ask if there were any songs he particularly liked. She said they listened to country music together when Brad was younger and he really liked Dierks Bentley's song "Home." Tony found a recording of the song and, in their next session, asked Brad if it was all right to play it (Brad shrugged *yes*). After a minute of listening, Brad hung his head and began to cry uncontrollably. Tony was taken aback, frozen for a few moments before turning the music off and asking, "What are you feeling?" Brad did not answer but continued to cry. When he calmed down he said, "I'd just like to go now," without looking at Tony. Tony said he could go but he wanted to talk about what happened in their next session. Brad said "Whatever," then left.

Tony realized that he may have somehow breached the trust in their relationship and that Brad felt unsafe. He asked Kumala what he had done wrong, or if there was something he could have done differently. Kumala first assured him that he had done the right thing by turning the music off, for leaving it on could have evoked even stronger emotions. She noted how music is processed differently than words, and that it can sneak into emotional centers without clients even knowing it is happening. She thought that the song "Home" might have brought up memories of happier times for Brad and that may have prompted him to think about how hard his life was now. The song might have served as a harsh reminder of how he was not home and how different the residential facility was from the house he grew up in.

She noted how the song did have the potential to become a point of reference for safely exploring Brad's sadness and grief, if done with care. Tony might have waited until Brad had calmed down and then just asked what it was about the song that made him cry, instead of pressing him to identify what he was feeling. He might also have built a sense of trust by approaching Brad directly rather than asking his mother which songs he liked.

Fostering Strengths, Control, and Resilience

Musical interaction, as with therapeutic play, builds resiliency by helping children express and manage their emotional world (Crenshaw et al., 2015). These interactions can foster a natural and immediate sense of connection, bring a client into the present moment, and involve his physical body in movement, which is an essential component of trauma recovery (van der Kolk, 2006). Children may be unable to speak directly about the issues weighing on them, yet be able to dance or move to the beat of a favorite song. Further, since children often sing spontaneously and unselfconsciously, they often are able to sing about what is on their mind, whether directly or indirectly, such as when Mike sang about the noisy cart.

Although catharsis, or the release of frozen emotion, is an important part of recovering from an intense shock or ordeal, it is not the end goal in processing trauma. Gaining a sense of control over emotional responses is recognized to be a vital part of recovery and requires going beyond catharsis (Loumeau-May, Seibel-Nicol, Hamilton, & Malchiodi, 2015). For healing to occur, it is critical that the child reexperience the emotional and body memories in a safe, therapeutic setting where they can be processed with a skilled therapist (Beck, D'Antonio, & Lyon, 2014).

Using music as a form of psychological first aid (NCTSN, n.d.-a) helps children recovering from trauma access hidden or blocked resources. This approach first requires stabilization of the situation so that the child is able to begin to cope with its aftermath. Once a sense of stability is achieved, interactive music can assist in establishing a sense of familiarity and safety, regulating emotions and responses, and reestablishing connections to people around them (Else, as cited in Stewart, 2010).

Children gravitate to music and find listening to or playing music satisfying and natural. Music makes them feel better, which reinforces their natural capacity for reparative play (Gil, 2017). Gil, in writing about posttraumatic play, says it provides children with "a distancing mechanism that allows children to 'own' their difficult memories gradually and to attempt to manage their underlying, often unspoken, concerns" (2017, p. 35). Music supports their instinct to express otherwise inaccessible emotions and work through them, thereby gaining a sense of mastery and control. A therapist who supports a child's musical play is able to see and hear the therapeutic process in action. The music offers a safe container for the child's intense feelings about the trauma, allowing him to proceed in therapy at his own pace. Children can safely reexperience overwhelmingly painful events and emotions, but with a different outcome: instead of being neglected or harmed, the child is cared for and comforted (Beck et al., 2014). The child's self-image changes from victim to survivor, and, beyond that, to hero or heroine (Lyon, 2005).

For teens, music is an easily accessed source of strength and pride: their musical choices are under their control and reflect who they are. Having the power to decide what music they like and want to listen to can enhance an adolescent's sense of identity as well as his sense of control over the world around him. This in turn can lead to an increase in resilience as he becomes better able to respond to the lingering effects of trauma.

VIGNETTE

Mandee was a 16-year-old girl who had been sexually abused by her uncle for over a year and was being counseled at school. During their second session together, her case worker, Andrea, asked Mandee what songs her mother sang to her when she was young, and she immediately answered, "You Are My Sunshine." Andrea responded by saying, "Yes! I know that song too. Can you remember how it goes?" Mandee started to sing the song in a very soft, subdued voice, and Andrea joined in, matching the soft quality of Mandee's voice. When they finished singing the first verse and chorus, they were both silent. After a short time, Andrea commented, "That one line, 'You make me happy when skies are gray,' is so positive. What do you think of it?" This led to a conversation about the words of the song. Mandee made an observation, "I think someone took my sunshine away," that Andrea found particularly revealing. She responded, "Someone did take your sunshine away, didn't they? What if we were to change the words to that line, and say, 'You can't take my sunshine away'?" Mandee looked directly at her and said, "Yes, I want to do that." Together they sang the new line, then the entire song, inserting the new words into it. The emotional tenor of the song changed, and Mandee visibly brightened, sitting up a little taller in her chair. For Mandee, "You Are My Sunshine" was a gateway to reconnecting to earlier, happier memories and to a time when she trusted the world; by singing her own lyrics she was able to assert her strength.

This vignette demonstrates how writing new lyrics to a favorite song allows the child to feel a sense of purpose and control, yet still maintain an emotional distance that does not threaten the sense of self. Another approach to lyric substitution is to write to one's past or future self. For example, an older child like Mandee who is grappling with the effects of sexual abuse can rewrite words to a favorite song as if she were writing them to herself before the abuse occurred. This may connect her to a part of herself that felt stronger, happier, and more in control. Substituting lyrics requires following a simple, clear structure to ensure that the client is comfortable with each step (see the sections on Changing Song Lyrics in "Recommendations for Practice" at the end of this chapter and Working with Song Lyrics in Chapter 2).

Another type of therapeutic music engagement that can help a child express the rhythms, dynamics, and landscapes of his inner emotional world is improvisation. Improvisation with traumatized children needs to be conducted with clear guidelines and intentions. Free improvisation can be scary for children who have suffered trauma; since they are unsure about what will happen next, they may fear both the unknown and losing control (Beer, 2011). This sense of fear may echo the original traumatic experience. Yet a child who successfully engages in improvisation in a supportive setting gains an experience of conquering his fear and surviving. It can build his tolerance for uncertainty, which is necessary in managing stress and anxiety. Since improvisation involves making musical choices, it can help transform feelings of helplessness and avoidance to feeling like being an active agent in one's life. Engaging in improvisational music can also be liberating in that it sparks spontaneity, which can help break a cycle of toxic or repetitive play (Gil, 2015).

Facilitating Emotion Regulation

As discussed in Chapter 3, emotion regulation refers to the child's ability to take in and process information and engage with the world in healthy ways (Scaer, 2014). Children who suffer from the effects of trauma often have difficulty regulating their emotional states, and early intervention that focuses on psychoeducation and managing feelings is crucial to healthy development (Kramer & Landolt, 2011). Music is one way for them to naturally engage in, learn, and initiate self-soothing behaviors, which in turn strengthen emotional coping strategies (Langdon, 2015). They become more spontaneous, and the flow of music gives them a sense of tension and release. An increase in tempo or dynamics can heighten emotions, while a decrease lessens a charged feeling. Traumatized children may need to relearn how to deal with swings in feelings and different sensations of anger, sadness, and fear. Music, with its structure, flexibility, emotional appeal, and natural anodynic effects, is one modality that holds much promise for clinical practice.

Not having a secure internal sense of control over emotions can be very upsetting to a child and can activate a cause–effect cycle that is difficult to break: when children feel out of control, they act out and reject support, and when they do not feel supported, they feel even more out of control (Siegel, 2012). Therapies such as dialectical behavior therapy (DBT) (Dimeff & Linehan, 2001) can be effective in helping older children and teens recognize patterns and begin to identify healthier ways to manage their emotions. However, younger children who have been traumatized may not be able to cognitively engage in this type of therapeutic interaction, due to their immaturity or the severity of the trauma suffered. Music, with its ability to bring a client into the present moment, a key aspect of DBT, can orient a child or teen to his current state of emotion while simultaneously offering a safe way to express and explore the sensations he is experiencing (Langdon, 2015).

Music can also provide a socially acceptable and satisfying way to express pent-up or unacknowledged rage that can be engendered by trauma (van der Kolk, 2017). It is not okay to act out against property or against other people, but it is okay to let out one's rage by beating a drum or crashing a cymbal. Making loud sounds can bring welcome relief. A child may also express anger in a song. One girl in therapy sang these improvised lyrics, her voice building to a dramatic crescendo as she reached the final phrase: "Go away, you're the reason I feel bad, Can't you see your meanness is making me sad, Why can't you be kind to me, I can't take it anymore, I can't believe what you did to me!"

Another point worth mentioning is how the aesthetic value of music relates to trauma. Trauma can cause children to lose their trust in the world and to see the world as a dangerous place. A child who has the experience of being transported by listening to or playing music may once again begin to find beauty in life. He may feel lifted out of himself in a way that brings joy and a sense of peace, no matter how transitory. Though he cannot change the original trauma, he can change the feelings accompanying the traumatic memory and open himself to more positive experiences.

Addressing the Dissociative Aspects of Trauma

Children at risk may have few coping options available to them. If they are not adequately protected, or cannot fight or flee the trauma, then their only options may be immobilization or dissociation. Immobilization occurs when a child withdraws or "freezes" and shuts down emotionally; the child ceases to respond to the outside world (Lyon et al., 2014). Some children try to escape the pain of trauma through dissociation, or by disconnecting their thoughts and feelings. Dissociation is a survival or coping skill, a kind of emotional numbing to deaden or block pain and trauma. The parts of the self associated with intolerable emotional pain become split off as the child tries to preserve a positive sense of self; there is a lack of personality integration (Bromberg, 2006).

Music can be extremely effective in helping children who have dissociative symptoms. Music works at a preverbal level and has the potential to access emotions directly, without having to go through cognitive filters (Austin, 2002). According to Birnbaum (2013), "Unresolved trauma 'cooks' internally; music gives it a voice" (Chapter 5, last paragraph). Although trauma can make a person feel like he has lost his sense of self, music can reintroduce a sense of reality, of being in the world. Engaging in a rhythmic experience through playing an instrument, such as vigorously beating a drum, or through movement, such as stamping one's feet firmly on the ground, can help a child feel his body and affirm his very existence. This corrective experience enables him to feel more connected both to himself and to the world at large.

Making music with others not only builds relationships, which is crucial in providing reparative experiences for children who have been traumatized, but is also a creative process that helps in healing. Children project their feelings into the music they create and, in so doing, reveal their inner worlds. By listening carefully and reflecting what a client does—answering a sung phrase, picking up on a tempo or rhythmic pattern—we communicate that we are hearing what the child is saying. By taking up a child's musical idea, the child feels understood and validated, and thus is more willing to take risks and express more feelings. By being "heard" via musical reflection, a child can bridge the rift between repressed emotion and social reality.

VIGNETTE

Amelia had been abused by her father from a very early age. At 26 months she was diagnosed with shaken baby syndrome, allegedly at the hands of her father. Although her overall development and cognitive abilities were normal, she had delays in gross motor development and poor self-regulation. Amelia was court-ordered to see her father with a supervisor once a week. After these visits she would come home agitated, aggressive, and clingy; she would stop eating solid food for days and had insomnia. When she did sleep she would wake up with nightmares and night terrors. She had episodes of extreme rage in which she beat up her dolls and slammed them against the walls, chewed on her own clothes and arms, and hit or bit her mother. After she had these outbursts, she would seek swaddling for deep pressure and used a pacifier for comfort.

Her mother reported that Amelia became withdrawn, depressed, and more detached from her caregivers after each visit with her father. She was afraid of anything unknown and had to be reassured if there were any changes to her routine. When Amelia felt comfortable, she was very social and bubbly and could be kind and loving. She loved music and dancing.

At the request of her mother, J.C.B. and another therapist began working with Amelia when she turned 3. Our main goal was to provide positive experiences in a safe and nurturing environment to help with self-regulation and coping with the trauma she had suffered, as well as the continuing trauma due to ongoing visitations with her father.

Amelia always brought a doll from home into the sessions, using this transitional object to provide psychological comfort. She played the role of mother for the doll, an indication of her strong identification with her own mother. At first, Amelia was hesitant to come into the therapy room and clung to her mother. She tended to reject invitations to participate in musical interactions. She was quiet and cautious and used gestures rather than words to express her likes or dislikes. Yet she showed curiosity about the instruments in the room and slowly began to engage with them, exploring both the large instruments (drum, xylophone) and the small rhythm instruments in the basket. She used her doll as a bridge to her own musical activity, by pretending to teach her "baby" to play the various instruments.

As Amelia's mother reported, we also observed that her withdrawn, clinging behavior was more intense after Amelia had weekend visitations with her father. She appeared to be extremely anxious and upset, crawling on her mother as if trying to merge with her for safety. Her play, both musical and dramatic, was characterized by a strong need to control the situation, which is typical of children who have suffered trauma. She frequently stopped us from playing or singing or told us to be quiet, though she often played loudly. No one could sing or play without her permission. When we offered her an idea, her tendency was to first reject it but then later take it up. Sometimes these rejections became playful musical call and response, for example, singing the word *no* back and forth between her and the therapists. By doing this we acknowledged her desire to resist, while showing her that interaction in music could be safe and fun. When we challenged her by deliberately not stopping, she often would smile and scold us in a teasing way. When she had not seen her father over the weekend, her emotional state was very different: she seemed relaxed and happy, ready to engage in musical experiences. At these times she cheerfully interacted with us and was more accepting of our interventions.

Amelia spontaneously made up stories that at first included just herself and her mother; she generally ignored our efforts to join in. She would ask her mother to speak for her rather than addressing us directly. It was clear that her identity and sense of safety were closely intertwined with her mother. We created music to support her stories and her interactions with her mother, giving her the space she needed to become more comfortable. Eventually she began to trust us; her shyness diminished, and she started talking to us directly.

We had a hunch that singing would offer Amelia an important creative outlet; however, this was hampered because she kept her pacifier in her mouth throughout most of the sessions. On the occasions when she did not use the pacifier, we discovered that she enjoyed singing and improvising vocally. She sang in tune and followed the rhythm/meter of the music, an expression of her innate musicality. At times she would engage in reciprocal singing with us, and related the action of the story through song, as in an opera, her voice strong and confident.

Sometimes she asked us to play a role in dramas that she directed. In her stories she often set up a private space just for her and her mother that we were not allowed to enter; she had a strong need to set her own boundaries. We respected her boundaries and sought other ways to participate in her storytelling. We found Disney and other children's songs, lullabies, and blues to be effective in supporting her musically. Through her musical play, Amelia was able to express her feelings and her creativity.

Amelia's participation in musical experiences reinforced her development in many different areas, including increasing her trust in herself and others; improving her self-confidence, feelings of self-worth and self-acceptance; identifying and validating her emotions; decreasing her levels of emotional stress and anxiety; and improving social interaction and social adjustment. Although Amelia was highly verbal, she was not able to use words to express her anger, fear, and sense of powerlessness. Music motivated her to reach out at her own pace, and to connect with others in ways that she found meaningful. In this way, it served to lessen her dissociative symptoms of detachment and emotional withdrawal and helped her gain a more integrated, healthy sense of self. Through singing and playing in a musical environment, she gained inner resources to help her cope with her difficult life circumstances.

GRIEF AND BEREAVEMENT

Losing a loved one is difficult for anyone yet is especially traumatic for children, who do not have the life experience or the fully developed emotional capacity to cope with the many challenges an unexpected, shocking, or dramatic loss brings. Once a vibrant and outwardly happy and engaged child, his loss of a loved one, whether sudden or after a long period of decline, brings forth new and potentially overwhelming feelings. While many children show resilience and bounce back from stressful events such as death or the divorce of their parents, others have more trouble coping (Cohen, Mannarino, & Deblinger, 2017). Symptoms of traumatic grief are more severe than what is considered normal grief responses and include having trouble sleeping, increased anxiety, fear of the dark, increased inability to focus while at school, withdrawal from friends, and not wanting to engage in activities they had previously enjoyed (Cohen, Mannarino, & Knudsen, 2004). In short, children suffering from traumatic grief often experience a change in their personalities, and how they respond to the world around them is altered in ways that, if untreated, can have enduring effects. They may come to believe they are unworthy of love and support, become angry, or avoid social situations they view as somehow threatening. The child's developmental level, support systems (or lack thereof), coping mechanisms, and internal resiliency determine the degree of intensity a loss will evoke (Cohen et al., 2004).

VIGNETTE

Cera, a 12-year-old child, resolutely and continuously claimed she was "fine" when asked how she was doing after her mother's sudden death. Cera's mother had been hit and killed by a drunk driver 6 months prior to Cera being seen by Mina, the school counselor. She was referred because she was not sleeping due to recurring nightmares about the accident, had difficulty sitting for more than 20 minutes in class, and had frequent angry outbursts directed toward the girls she had been close friends with prior to her mother's death. Mina knew Cera had a passion for music: she sang in the school choir and played the viola in the orchestra. Mina wondered if focusing on Cera's love of music would create rapport and help her feel at ease.

In their first one-to-one session, Cera came into the room, sat down, and said to Mina, "I really don't want to be here. I don't know what good it will do." Mina told Cera they did not have to talk about anything in particular, but that she had heard Cera had been having some trouble in class and she was there to support her. She then asked Cera what songs she most liked listening to. Cera responded, "I dunno, there are a lot." She then listed several songs she had on her playlist, and Mina suggested they listen to a couple of them together. Cera agreed, and Mina found two of the songs on her phone and played them. One of them was Katy Perry's "Roar." Mina pulled up the lyrics and, after listening to the song, read some of them. She noted that the words were about becoming independent and vocal, roaring like a lion with strength and confidence. She asked Cera what she thought of the words to the song, and she responded, "Well, I think I am roaring these days but it's not because I feel strong." With some gentle prompting by Mina, she continued, "I am just so mad. I don't know what to do. Nothing is the same." Cera became quiet, and together they sat in silence for a few moments. Realizing that pushing Cera for more disclosure could have detrimental effects, Mina closed the session after listening to another, less emotive song on Cera's playlist.

Mina realized that, in choosing this song, Cera was acknowledging the pain and confusion she was experiencing in an indirect, symbolic way. The song "Roar" has a positive message yet can also speak to a lion's roar of anger or aggression. She felt Cera was allowing herself to feel anger yet also holding onto the hope that her roar could become a sound of strength again.

In their third session, Mina was surprised when Cera chose Fauré's "Requiem," apparently because her choir at school was learning two movements of the work. Mina asked what the requiem was about, and Cera explained it was about dying and finding peace. Mina was struck by the direct parallel to Cera's life yet did not verbalize this. She found a version and played the first movement. After it ended she said to Cera, "This is a beautiful piece of music. It sounds sad and also hopeful all at once." Cera was very still, her hair covering her face as she looked downward. Mina saw Cera was softly crying and handed her some tissues but did not say anything. After a few minutes Cera wiped her eyes and said, "I just miss her so much." Mina responded, "Yes, I can only imagine how much you miss her. What do you miss most?" From there Cera began to talk about her mother, about her struggle to talk to her friends, and how lonely she felt.

This session marked a breakthrough for Cera. The "Requiem" allowed Mina to experience grief alongside Cera without having to force a discussion. The music seemed to embody feelings of intense sadness yet also had an upward, soaring type of movement. She continued to meet with Mina, listen to music, and talk about how to cope with what she was feeling. There was no immediate or dramatic improvement in Cera's engagement in school, yet each day seemed to bring a stronger sense of balance and connection to her friends and to her studies.

Music captures and expresses intense human emotions like grief and sadness and allows us to safely experience these emotions. In Cera's case, the music allowed her to feel these emotions without having to verbalize what she felt. But once the emotions were brought up, it was easier to talk about them. The act of listening to music together strengthened the therapeutic relationship and created a natural and safe rapport between therapist and client.

VIGNETTE

Rhea, a 6-year-old girl, had lost her baby sister 2 months prior to my (L.E.B.) meeting her. Rhea's sister was born with severe physical impairments and died when she was 14 months old. When this happened, Rhea stopped talking and shied away from all physical contact. She was referred to a creative arts bereavement camp for children by the hospice social worker who had worked with the family. I met Rhea on the first day of camp; she stayed outside of the opening music circle and watched most of the activities that went on, choosing not to actively participate. Staff members invited her to engage but did not overly encourage her, letting her make the decision as to when to step into a group experience.

On the second day of camp, Rhea came to the music circle and sat with the other children. She did not make eye contact, but when a drum was passed around and each child was prompted to beat as they said their names, she beat the drum twice but did not say her name. The two beats were quick and steady, reflective of the syllables in her name. This was a start, a benign way for her to be part of the group, yet not give up the power of her silence. This activity was repeated every day when camp started and Rhea engaged in it, each day playing a little more and following prompts to "play what your favorite color is," "play to sound out something we don't know about you" (this was followed by an optional invitation to share what that "something" was), and "play what you are feeling today." I noted that Rhea became increasingly comfortable with this drum game and began to laugh with the other children when they said something funny or pulled a silly face. This repeated activity offered a secure way for Rhea to feel playful and comfortable interacting with others.

SUMMARY

Feelings of helplessness, uncontrollable emotions, lack of trust, and underachievement are hallmarks of traumatized children's behavior (Robarts, 2003, 2014). The disempowerment and loss of trust in adults who were supposed to protect them is profound and can be difficult to regain, even in a safely regulated therapeutic environment. As seen with Rhea, with the introduction of simplified, clear musical games or interactions, children can gain control over emotional expression and feel a sense of power and achievement. The dyadic interaction between therapist and client can lead to a greater capacity to tolerate healthy relationships (Gil, 2017). There are many ways a psychotherapist can use music to bridge a therapeutic relationship or help a client connect with his inner emotional life; what is most important is to always work within the client's comfort zone and to keep it an activating and fulfilling experience.

The ultimate goal in working with children recovering from trauma is to help them regain a sense of security and to feel whole. Finding ways to effectively and developmentally treat trauma is essential in helping a child learn how to manage emotions, forge positive relationships, and grow into a balanced and stable adult. This chapter explored how music, when sensitively and intentionally used, can help a child cope with the effects of trauma, explore emotions safely, and interact with others in a natural and satisfying way.

RECOMMENDATIONS FOR PRACTICE

As discussed in this chapter, guidelines include establishing a foundation of trust and security by being at ease, giving clear verbal instructions, letting the child know there are no expectations for performance, and having a "let's just see what happens" attitude. Before bringing one of the following exercises into a session, be sure to try them out on your own. Become familiar with how *you* respond to the instructions and find the best way for you to engage your client musically while being your authentic self. Also, experiment with any instrument you want to bring into the therapy room. Make sure you are comfortable playing all of them in a variety of ways.

Listening to Music Together

- The example of Brad's response to "Home" shows how identifying a song that might have meaning for a child and playing it for him can loosen deep-seated emotions. Often, children do not know what they are feeling, or are feeling many different things simultaneously, and cannot find the words that would define or articulate their feelings.
- In some cases the therapist can wait on seeking verbal feedback ("How does it feel?") and allow the child to choose whether to let the song fade into silence or to respond verbally.
- There are also times when no verbal processing is needed. Allowing Brad to cry for a while, and then asking if he wanted to talk about something else, helped move him from an emotionally charged situation to safer ground. In this way, a therapist can build trust and become a partner in listening to music.

Karaoke

- Sing along to a song, karaoke-style. By listening to a client's favorite song (given language and violence parameters for the lyrics), you will be tuned into the musical culture of your clients. One way to build upon a child's natural inclination to sing along to favorite songs is

to bring a song into a session that the client identified as one of his favorites.
- Talk with your client or his caregiver to find out what songs he likes. Be sure that the child is comfortable with the caregiver's recommendations.
- Choose two songs, find the lyrics (*www.chordie.com* is a wonderful resource), and print them out before your next session. Having the lyrics typed out for older children gives them something to focus on while engaging in the music and also serves as a point of reference should you want to change some of the lyrics (addressed in the following section).
- Have the child choose one of the prepared songs.
- Play the song and listen to it with your client. Depending on the age of the child, you may want to either talk about the lyrics or play the song again and sing along to it.
- Play the song and sing along. With a younger client who is not cognitively able to reflect on lyrics, sing along to the song and, if your client starts dancing, dance or move in a way that supports the way he is moving. Try not to be inhibited about singing or moving to the song, especially if your client is freely singing or dancing. This is not about performing, but rather doing what comes naturally for both the child *and* you. Singing and/or dancing together is a bonding agent and opens a pathway to be more spontaneous and playful with a client in a structured and boundaried way.

Changing Song Lyrics

This is an immediate and clear way to open up your client's response to the song as well as to deepen your therapeutic relationship.

- With older children who may be reluctant to sing in front of someone else, look at the lyrics together and open a conversation about them. Phrases to use can include, "What do you like best about what the song says?" or "Have you ever felt that way?"
- You can also point out striking features of the song to talk about: Does it have a unique rhythm or melody? Does the melody reflect the title of the song? Is it fast, slow, or does it change tempos? All parts of a song can be talked about. This engages your client in a discussion that is

not directly about him yet speaks to who he is, his preferences, likes, and dislikes.
- If a song has a specific feeling attached to it, the lyrics or musical feel can serve as an oblique way to explore the child's inner emotional landscape.
- Keep the new lyrics simple, for example, by choosing a familiar folk song like "Home on the Range." It is surprising how many teenagers know this song and will join in singing it and finding new words to put to it.
- After listening to a preferred song together, suggest writing new lyrics to the child's past or future self.
- Some songs lend themselves to writing completely new lyrics. For example, "My Favorite Things" (from *The Sound of Music* by Rodgers and Hammerstein) invites people to think about what they like most.
  - Identify favorite people, events, foods, or memories as a way to connect with positive aspects of a child's history and life.
  - Write them down, ordering them in a way that fits the melody, and sing them; the song becomes a celebration of the unique person that is your client. No one else in the world will have those specific things to sing about.
  - Typing the lyrics out and presenting them to the client as a transitional object when terminating therapy can create a tangible affirmation of his strengths.
- Certain song forms, such as the 12-bar blues, evoke different kinds of lyrics. Starting with a phrase such as "Woke up this morning, and I was feeling _____" invites a person to reflect on his day and what was important and opens the door to bring up more "blue" emotions such as sadness and hardship. It is important to allow time for a client to respond without guiding him as to what to say, and to accept whatever ideas the client offers.

Spontaneous Songs

Singing can take many different forms: it may be a known and preferred song; a simple, improvised melody sung with words or syllables, hummed or whistled; or a chant of a repeated phrase that picks up on the child's own words or actions, or nonsense syllables.

- Try making up a song about what your client is doing, or perhaps about a favorite animal or food.
- Connecting the song with something meaningful or immediate will bring him into the experience more fully.
- Creating a steady rhythm and using repetition are important steps to include. As mentioned earlier, a steady beat or rhythm gives a sense of security, while repeating phrases or melodies increases a sense of mastery. Incorporating a rocking or other rhythmic movement can have a soothing effect and contribute to the sense of engagement.
- Keep the song moving at a predictable tempo. This creates a sense of flow that is an important aesthetic component of music. Even very young children respond to a song that is aesthetically pleasing! The flow of music also provides an inward sense of continuity that is often lost when a child is coping with the aftermath of trauma (Turry, 2002).

Instrument Play

Allowing a client to play and explore instruments unfamiliar to him can yield important information about how he approaches new experiences. In this case, having instruments available for the child to play independently of the therapist can have strong therapeutic value.

- Bring out one or two instruments each session that you are confident your client does not have experience in playing. An African drum such as the djembe, or a more recent North American creation, the tubano, are examples of larger drums. There are many world instruments that could serve you here, as outlined in Chapter 2.
- Have your client choose an instrument to explore.
- Together, find different ways to play it.
- Play one of your client's favorite songs and encourage him to play the instrument along to it. You can provide support by playing a smaller percussion instrument such as an egg shaker or maraca.
- Instrument play with familiar and well-liked instrument: Playing an instrument can be like spending time with an old friend. Children may express clear preferences and have strong feelings about certain instruments. Offer at least two different instruments—more, if a child can handle a wider selection without becoming distracted or overwhelmed. Giving choices allows a child to exercise control. Having time during

a therapy session to play a favorite instrument may bring comfort to a child and foster creativity as he explores new ways of playing.

Sounding Emotions

The purpose of this exercise is to identify along with your client emotions that someone, not necessarily the client, might feel. Using two hand drums, such as djembes or bongos (one for the client and one for the therapist), play the drums using your hands and then experiment with how to play what each emotion might sound like. This exercise can lead to a sense of control over varying emotions. For example, a child who has difficulty expressing anger might find it easier to play the drum loud and fast, while another child might want to play softly to sound out what sadness feels like. The choice of whether to verbally process this work is up to the therapist's discretion.

- Set the drums up in the therapy room so they are the only instruments there.
- Show your client several ways to play the drums; for example, by playing with a flat hand in the middle you get a deeper, louder sound, or by playing with fingers on the edge you get a sharper, lighter tone.
- Introduce the exercise by speaking with your client about emotions and how they can be hard to talk about. Or, if your client is resistant or unable to express himself easily with words, you may offer photographs or simple pictures of mad, sad, and glad faces.
- Ask the client to choose either mad, sad, or glad to play on the drums.
- Start playing a steady beat and ask your client to start playing what the emotion feels like. By establishing a predictable rhythmic pulse, you will give the experience boundaries and a sense of safety. Resist the urge to mirror how your client is playing so that he has a "safe sound," the steady beat, to return to if he feels overwhelmed.
- When you have worked through one or more emotions, gently explore what the experience was like for him; you can also highlight aspects of his playing, for example, "I heard how your music started slow but got faster when you played 'mad.' What do you think happened there?"
- After several repetitions or when your client is ready to move on to another level, bring in concepts relevant to the child. For example, for a client who has nightmares, you could introduce "peace," "pretty sunset," or "falling stars" to play.

Improvisation

Finding a theme and improvising on it can be a freeing experience for a client who is used to holding himself tightly in and avoiding emotions associated with the trauma he suffered. Improvising in music connects the body, spirit, imagination, and social and cognitive parts of the self; the creative act of making music can make a child feel more alive.

- If a child is processing grief, engaging in an improvisation that alternates between two emotions, such as happy and sad, can be empowering.
- The client chooses an instrument while you give instructions that when you play one instrument (e.g., the cowbell), it signals the music should sound happy, and when you play another (e.g., a small xylophone) the music should switch to sounding sad.
- After a few repetitions of this your client will probably want to be the one controlling how to play—let him do this while you follow his instructions.
- Choose two other emotions to contrast. These could be happy–mad and mad–sad, or for clients who are older, other emotional opposites such as frustrated–easygoing, ashamed–proud, or afraid–confident.

Creating Playlists of Thematically Clustered Songs

Identifying a theme that supports a client's strengths is important here and could include something the client is good at or particularly likes. We recommend avoiding themes centered on anger or sadness as these may serve to intensify a client's feelings of grief or of being angry. Delving into strong emotional centers when listening to songs can activate unexpected responses, such as what Brad experienced. These clustered songs can become playlists for the client to listen to.

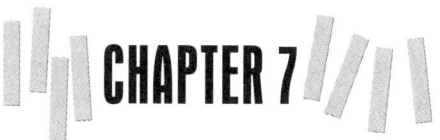

CHAPTER 7

Children with Behavioral, Emotional, and Communication Disorders

Children who experience debilitating psychiatric problems think, behave, and experience emotions in often unpredictable ways (American Academy of Child and Adolescent Psychiatry, 2009). It is estimated that 3–5% of the children in the United States have attention-deficit/hyperactivity disorder (ADHD), 1–4% of children between the ages of 9 and 17 have conduct disorder (CD), one in 10 of every child or adolescent in the United States experiences major depression, and one in 59 children under the age of 10 has autism spectrum disorder (ASD). A 2016 study found that nearly 28% of children with ASD engage in behaviors that can lead to self-injury; whether in classrooms, residential facilities, or hospitals, children with self-injurious behaviors do not function well (Soke et al., 2016). Many children with these and other diagnoses have comorbid conditions, making treatment even more complex. For example, as many as 80% of children diagnosed with ADHD also have at least one other disorder such as anxiety or depression, and up to 50% have two or more issues that intersect and affect them (Pliszka, 2015). Success in treatment for these children includes reducing frequent explosive outbursts, thereby increasing their ability to communicate basic needs, and helping them develop the prosocial skills necessary to have friends.

Serious psychological problems in children take myriad behavioral, cognitive, and emotional forms. These can result in challenging behaviors that cause high levels of stress for families and caregivers. Doctors and clinicians must rely upon observation, family history, and physical evaluations to assess symptomology and properly treat a child exhibiting acute responses. Whether the child's problems are rooted in the genetic, neurological, cognitive, or emotional realm, treatment of high-incidence disorders often focuses on teaching appropriate behaviors and helping the child learn how to interact in a manner that is positive and socially acceptable (DeKlyen & Greenberg, 2016).

Interventions may combine psychotherapy, medication, and psychosocial rehabilitation, including, for example, reward-centered treatment such as applied behavior analysis (ABA), cognitive-behavioral therapy (CBT), acceptance and commitment therapy (ACT) to increase flexibility (Swain, Hancock, Dixon, Koo, & Bowman, 2013), and psychotropic and antianxiety drugs (Compton et al., 2014). Medication may not always be an effective long-term remedy due to unpredictable results, side effects, and nonresponse rates (Compton et al., 2014; Cornacchio, Bry, Sanchez, Poznanski, & Comer, 2017; McKay, Abramowitz, & Storch, 2017). Research findings indicate nonpharmacological approaches can, in many cases, be effective (Morano et al., 2017). As such, psychosocial, behavioral, multimodal, and creative arts approaches are often important sources of ongoing care.

There has been considerable support for the use of creative arts in treatment (Malchiodi, 2015; Robarts, 2014; Porges, 2011). The inherent characteristics of music—its rhythm, repetition, and power to evoke strong emotions—can make it a significant part of a treatment plan when utilized by a sensitive and attuned therapist. This chapter addresses how music can be incorporated in therapy to address symptoms that are common across disorders. It also includes a special section on ASD, an area where there has been more research regarding music as a therapeutic intervention.

MUSIC AS A SUPPORTIVE INTERVENTION

Music may provide a valuable connection with a child who is difficult to reach or resistant to contact. Since a musical experience can be entered into without direct contact with another person or reliance on language, it can bypass negative patterns of interaction and allow for new forms of relationship to emerge.

Current trends in treatment focus on the importance of recognizing the child's capacity to develop his own resiliency and ability to self-regulate (Kinniburgh, Blaustein, Spinnazola, & van der Kolk, 2017), and with music, a therapist can take a strengths-based approach. Tapping into a child's musical abilities by playing or listening to music together builds relationships in a way that is proximal yet nonthreatening, interactive yet also independent. The child and the therapist work together in a space of communicative play: cognition is activated, and the child needs to control his behaviors so he can play and sing effectively. In a group setting, the overall sound of the music depends on everyone's full involvement. For children with substantial emotional or behavioral issues, music making can bring about a sense of pleasure and confidence that may be an unusual and very satisfying experience.

Music making also provides an opportunity to offer choices to children who are often not able to make choices for themselves. Making decisions is a necessary part of creating resiliency and a healthy identity (Duarte, 2017). Asking a child if he wants to hear music that is fast or slow, or loud or soft (musical elements of tempo and dynamics described in Chapter 1) is empowering and builds confidence. Creating such occasions for making choices is possible both in individual and group settings.

Facilitating Language

Music and singing can facilitate both the production and comprehension of language for all children, and can be especially helpful for children with verbal delays. Children typically learn song lyrics by filling in single words, usually at the end of a line (e.g., "Twinkle, twinkle little _____" and the child fills in "star"). By singing a familiar song and pausing before the last word, the therapist invites the child to complete the line. If necessary, the therapist can provide prompts, for example, by making the first sound of the word and waiting to see if the child will attempt to sing the entire word. Slowing the pace to fit the child's responses allows him time to process and produce the needed word; recorded music may be too fast and therefore less effective. Once a child is able to fill in a single word, the therapist can provide many opportunities to build the child's language production by leaving space for two words, short phrases, and then longer phrases.

Songs that reinforce concepts such as colors, body parts, or clothing help to build awareness and vocabulary. You can encourage the child to label body parts by pointing to his hand, foot, nose, etc., and asking him to fill in the word: for example, "This is my _____." A song can ask, "What color is your shirt?" Adding more detail helps build greater perception and language: it has short sleeves, perhaps, or white buttons, or black stripes. Virtually any concept or topic can be put into a song, which children often find more engaging than a spoken lesson. You can borrow a melody from a familiar song or create your own. Simply singing back and forth between two notes in a sing-song manner may stimulate response in a child.

In addition to concrete items, or things they can see or touch, children can label abstract ideas such as emotions or concepts that are not immediately present. Songs that focus on specific categories work well:

- "When you are hungry, what do you like to eat?"
- "What do you wear in different kinds of weather?"
- "What do you do after school?"
- "What other movements can you do besides jumping?"

These kinds of songs build comprehension as the child initiates a verbal or musical response.

Supporting Organized Communications and Interactions

Children with serious mental health problems are often unable to organize their verbal or behavioral responses to people and situations in order to communicate their wants, needs, and impulses (DeKleypen & Greenberg, 2016). This type of disorganization is known to be a precursor to antisocial and avoidant behaviors later in childhood and into adolescence (DeKleypen & Greenberg, 2016). Related characteristics of children who present with high levels of disorganization are difficulties with eye gaze, repetitive speech or vocal patterns, low affect, and behaviors that create safety issues and disruptive environments (Porges, 2011).

Music offers the child a means to experience what it is like to be organized through playing instruments and engaging in focused listening experiences. These activities require a degree of self-organization and can move children toward a healthier engagement in life (Ford, 2017). The following vignette shows how basic rhythms may be used to help organize a child's thinking and interactions when verbal attempts have failed.

VIGNETTE

Dawn began seeing Rudy, a 3-year-old child with Down syndrome, in play therapy. He had limited verbal language abilities but had well-developed receptive language capabilities for his age. His mother reported that he fell into fits of screaming or pinching when he was unable to make his needs known. His outbursts were explosive and destructive to the people and things around him, and his parents were reaching a point of high frustration. When Dawn first met Rudy, she showed him a medium-sized frame drum and a mallet, and demonstrated how to play it fast, slow, loud, and soft. When she handed the drum and mallet to him, Rudy began enthusiastically beating the drum. Dawn matched his tempo and dynamics on another drum, and he looked up at her and laughed loudly. She noticed how his drumming was steady. She felt this stable, rhythmic beating reflected a capacity for internal organization that was not evident in how he responded to the world. They spent much of their session time together playing in this manner, with Rudy often shouting "Yeah!" and laughing with abandon. His parents marveled at how he could play for up to 10 minutes, as well as at his ability to change his tempo and dynamics to match Dawn's changes.

After three sessions, Dawn met with Rudy's mother and related her observations that his drumming was strong, organized, and flexible. He was responsive to rhythms, able to make sustained eye contact, and take pleasure in the interactions with his therapist. When playing music with her he could respond to new rhythms or sounds she introduced. He also laughed and whooped whenever she played back some of his sounds and rhythms. Dawn talked about how this might carry over into his daily life. As a result, his mother began walking or marching and chanting in time to the steps, singing about what Rudy was doing in a confident voice, and praising his drumming abilities to others when he was within earshot as part of their everyday routines.

Encouraging Prosocial Behavior

Group settings are particularly useful for fostering prosocial behaviors because working to play together in a group creates an environment where children are navigating proximity to others. For example, a therapist or educator can provide a small percussion instrument (like an egg shaker or small hand drum) for the children to pass around in a circle with instructions to stop playing when the therapist stops the recorded music and pass the instrument to the person next to them. The social micro-interactions required for a child to engage in this activity include making eye contact, waiting his turn, playing the instrument for the time indicated, and communicating with the person next to him. The gestalt of this experience helps "form the basis of the child's ability to develop more complex and coherent ways of being with significant others" (Hart, 2017, p. 59).

Music groups foster cooperative behavior with peers. A child who is bullying others in school, for example, may be carefully encouraged to play or sing a song together with peers; he may also solo with the support of the group or write his own verse to a favorite song, which would then be sung by the group. These are concrete ways to help a child develop empathy, strengthen self-awareness, and increase positive social interactions (Trevarthen & Panksepp, 2017). Collaborating with peers on creating a musical experience involving imagery (see Chapter 2), such as what it might sound like to climb a mountain, is another way to nurture and encourage listening to others and being part of a team effort. Talking about what it is like to see mountains, or envisioning climbing a mountain, can lead into a structured musical sequence of starting out, walking uphill, getting tired, reaching the top, then walking back down. Using instruments such as djembe drums to establish a steady rhythmic pattern to demonstrate walking, getting louder and slower to symbolize getting tired, playing faster and lighter to express the excitement of reaching the top, then moving back into the walking pattern, is an imaginative form of play. Inherent in this activity is an experience of working together, a sense of accomplishment (in reaching the top), and satisfaction in returning to the starting point. There are also therapeutic possibilities for group discussion or creative expression in each of these stages. Finding ways to engage the musical impulse of a child in a group setting can have surprising and beneficial outcomes.

VIGNETTE

Brock was a 7-year-old child with severe impulse-control problems that greatly affected his ability to participate in classroom learning activities, communicate, and play with his peers. His mother brought him to a music group with children who were more socially capable than he was, hoping that he would learn other modes of interacting. For several weeks Brock did not sit in the circle with the other children. He was not refusing to participate but, given his difficulties with impulse control, was simply unable to sit still long enough. The group leader worked with Brock's aide to give her some ideas on how to help him during the music sessions. The aide learned to sing his name as Brock walked by her as he circled the room. In one session, when she sang his name with a rhythmic drive to it ("Brock-Brock-BROCK!"), he stopped, looked at her, and laughed. After repeating this several times, she began singing the "The ABC Song" to him (his favorite song) but in a tempo that matched the music that was being played with the other children in the group. Smiling and laughing, Brock went over and sat in her lap and started to sing along, matching the tempo, dynamics, and rhythm of the group's music.

Music helps children develop inner resources of control. Engaging in musical play required Brock to attend to "The ABC Song" and to how the aide was singing it to him. He needed to control his impulses to be able to create music that was satisfying. Although he remained at the periphery of the group, he was connected to the music that the group was playing and experienced an intrinsic motivation to join in. In turn, this gave him a sense of enjoyment and involvement with others. By being mindful of his comfort zone and his tolerance for somatic arousal, his aide was able to work with his desire to sing the song and connect him to the group's social environment. This helped Brock to break his pattern of behavior and become more involved in a playful and meaningful exchange (Goldstein & Ogden, 2017).

Regulating High Levels of Emotion

Children experiencing high levels of behavioral, mental, and social distress typically have difficulty regulating their emotions; finding ways to increase awareness and develop management strategies are important to their growth and development (Powers, Etkin, Gyurak, Bradley, & Jovanovic, 2015). Music as a form of individual as well as group expression can help decrease dysregulation when focused in a therapeutic manner. Therapists can work with children by sounding out strong emotions in musical play and using strategies for managing them. This requires focused attention as well as an awareness of what the child is capable of handling. Children who have difficulty regulating emotion require simple musical interactions to avoid overstimulating or overwhelming them. For example, you may want to introduce a drumming activity by first demonstrating various ways to play the drum, how beating it in different areas yields different sounds, and how to play softly as well as loudly, and fast as well as slow.

VIGNETTE

Autumn, who was 4 years old, had a debilitating anxiety disorder that manifested in refusals to leave her home, a fear of adults, and sleep difficulties. In therapy, she initially avoided any direct interaction with me (L. E. B.) and did not respond to verbal prompts or questions. She tested at a normal range of intelligence, and I viewed her reluctance to interact as her habitual means of coping with a new person and adjusting to a new situation. I wanted to build a relationship with her that was nonthreatening, and music provided an indirect way of connecting with her.

Autumn spent the first two sessions moving around the periphery of the therapy room humming to herself. I felt that her movements and sounds were helping her self-soothe and gave her the time and space to become comfortable in the room. After a while, I mirrored her humming and matched the pitch vocally and on the guitar. However, as soon as I found the right note, Autumn quickly switched to another key. When she started humming again, I matched her pitch and this time she lapsed into silence. This pattern continued several more times: she stopped humming when I attempted to join in. I knew that children like Autumn may not immediately respond to therapy, so I stopped trying to engage her in this way and waited to see what would happen.

In our third session, I spontaneously started singing "Ring Around the Rosy" as Autumn came into the therapy room. When she got to the middle of the room she started singing, "Ashes, ashes, we all fall down." I repeated this line and sat down when I sang "fall down." Autumn laughed and sat down with me. I said, "Should we try falling down?" and she nodded her head energetically. We stood up, sang the song again, and this time collapsed to the floor at the end of it, laughing together at the silliness of it all. I whispered, "Should we stay on the floor, or should we get up again and this time try dancing around?" Autumn whispered back, "Let's dance around." So we got up, sang the song, and at the end, instead of "Ashes, ashes, we all fall down," we sang, "Ashes, ashes, we all dance around." After a brief time of dancing, I sang, "Ashes, ashes, let's all sit down," which we enacted. I then asked Autumn what else we could do at the end of the song, and she said, "Fly like a bird." So we flew like birds, then sat down.

This experience was moving for me, for it was the first time Autumn and I engaged in an authentic, playful interaction. For a few minutes, she was not a child with a disabling anxiety disorder, but simply a child playing. The structure of the song allowed us to sing, dance, and fly. It also gave her the opportunity to practice recovering quickly from abrupt changes, something that was typically difficult for her to do. Catharsis, or building tension and moving toward release, is a natural musical phenomenon that can be helpful for children like Autumn in their treatment process.

Identifying Emotions

The ability to identify one's emotions is a fundamental component of social communication, and the first step in learning how to manage and express them in a positive and healthy way. A child who is aware of his own feelings is better able to understand these feelings in others. Difficulty in recognizing and naming emotions can result in poor self-regulation and interpersonal skills (Eisenberg et al., 2016; Trevarthen, Aitken, Papoudi, & Robarts, 1998).

Many factors contribute to a child's emotional competence, including age, culture, temperament, and previous negative experiences. Recent research (e.g., Javdani et al., 2017) found that teens with posttraumatic stress disorder (PTSD) and CD have trouble correctly identifying facial expressions. Being able to identify facial expressions is "a central mechanism for communicating emotional states and is crucial for the development of adaptive social functioning" (Javdani et al., 2017, p. 1). The authors show that teens with PTSD often confused anger with being fearful, and teens with CD had difficulty recognizing sadness.

Some children with difficult problems may lack empathy or, due to their inability to recognize typical emotions, are callous in their responses. One of the goals of therapy with such individuals, therefore, is for the client to be able to learn what different emotions feel like and look like. Music, with its natural emotional expression, can be an effective modality to facilitate this process. When used sensitively and carefully, music can evoke and embody various emotions (Brown, 2017). For example, using a picture of a sad face and combining it with music that has a mournful tone and impression (e.g., Barber's "Adagio") can, with prompting and encouragement, increase recognition. Identifying emotions during the safety of the therapy session can lead to more generalized identification of emotional expression, as shown in the case of Kimmi below.

VIGNETTE

Kimmi, a 13-year-old girl, had recently been diagnosed with PTSD and CD following the death of her younger sister in a home marked by domestic violence. Kimmi was removed from her parents' care and placed with an aunt and uncle, Tracy and Dan, and their two children in a stable and loving home. She had to change schools and a social worker was assigned to work with her. Despite Tracy's efforts to help her recover from all this trauma, Kimmi began acting out and became increasingly combative. She began to skip school and was seen several times smoking cigarettes with a group of older teens. She refused to talk about any of the traumas she had suffered in her sessions with the social worker. They often ended up discussing movies, music, and happenings at school, not moving beyond the surface of her experiences. Things at home were deteriorating; Kimmi was becoming physically aggressive with her younger cousins, and Tracy and Dan did not know how much longer they could have her in their house. Tracy noted how Kimmi seemed out of touch with her emotions as well as those of others around her. The only time Kimmi seemed to recognize emotion was when she listened to music. Tracy said, "Well, she seems to be okay when she listens to music. When a song is about something happy, she smiles and dances around, but when it is about something sad, like a break-up, she looks sad." The social worker had not known this about Kimmi and referred her to Irene, a child psychologist specializing in the use of creative arts. After taking a detailed history, Irene opened her first session by playing a classical piece by Mozart and moving to the music using scarves alongside Kimmi. When the music ended, Kimmi said, "Can we do that again?" Irene put on another piece of music that had a happy, upbeat tempo and again they moved around the room, laughing together at some of the movements they made.

Irene started and ended each of their 10 sessions with movement to music, varying the pieces to either fit Kimmi's mood or to introduce a different mood. After the first session, Kimmi started to talk about the music and how it made her feel. She also offered explanations for why she initiated certain movements, demonstrating to Irene that she was developing the capacity to identify her emotions and was also becoming aware of her bodily responses. This work laid a foundation for Kimmi to understand how and why emotions affected her, and to begin to verbalize her thoughts and feelings. Tracy noted that Kimmi's presence at home was less volatile and more interactive.

Creating Routines and Facilitating Transitions

Routines provide structure to our day and help us navigate our lives. They provide a means to move smoothly from one activity to another without the anxiety of having to make too many decisions and help us feel safe. When routines become embedded with special meaning they become rituals, which give us comfort and security. Yet sometimes children become overly dependent on routines or see them as confining. Children with severe ASD or obsessive–compulsive disorder (OCD) can have a rigid need for sameness or, conversely, for children with oppositional deficient disorder (ODD), an aversion to routine and ritual. If routines vary, even slightly, they can be a source of extreme anxiety for some children, while others resist predictability and constancy. The repetition inherent in music, as rhythms and melodies repeat in a predictable way, can provide a feeling of security in children who have a strong need for sameness.

Transitions are often a time of anxiety and even chaos, particularly for those children with pathological behavioral and emotional issues. Experts agree that children tend to feel most comfortable when expectations are clear, and they know what is going to happen next and what they are supposed to do (Stormshak, DeVargas, & Cárdenas, 2017). Creating consistency and "promoting structure, predictability, and follow-through in children's environments is key" (Cornacchio et al., 2017, p. 444). We saw in Chapter 3 how music could be used to cue children when moving to and from environments such as the lunchroom. When working with children who have severe problems, there are other approaches for using music, such as using a hand drum or bell to call attention or create transition rituals between events or activities. This helps the children focus on an environmental stimulus and less on the expectation of compliance inherent in using verbal instruction alone. Children who are living in a residential or inpatient unit can take responsibility for transitions. Being assigned the job of "drum player" when it is time to go to music or art period can be a source of pride for a child. The child must be able to demonstrate a level of self-control and self-awareness to go to where the drum is kept at the appropriate time, ask for the drum, play it in a moderate dynamic, and return it.

Music can also help children with everyday routines such as going to sleep. Bedtime can be a time of stress for many children, especially those with deep-seated anxieties and behavioral challenges. For younger children, bedtime can be especially challenging, for it is difficult for them to suddenly lie down in a darkened room and be alone. Creating a song with the child that has a simple, familiar tune and writing lyrics that address the child's source of anxiety and offer solace helps him feel some control over this time of day. Lullabies and lullaby-like songs are particularly effective with young children in helping them become calmer (Loewy et al., 2013). The therapist must be sensitive to the chronological and/or developmental age of the child, but many younger children respond to songs that have a lullaby feel to them when presented in the context of going to sleep. Taking a familiar song such as "Twinkle, Twinkle, Little Star" and creating lyrics that a younger child can learn and sing to himself empowers him. Using the tune of the song, a child who fears going to sleep could sing,

> When it's time to go to bed
> I'll feel safe and rest my head
> As I close my eyes to sleep
> I can have good dreams to keep
> Now it's time to go to bed
> I'll feel safe and rest my head.

Should you experiment with this strategy, we recommend you sing the song with the child several times or repeat it in successive sessions so it becomes increasingly familiar. The child may come to think of this song as "his," giving him a sense of ownership and comfort. Creating simple, soothing songs can help to ease nighttime transitions as well as others that may be stressful for the child.

While some children thrive on schedules and consistency, others are averse to expectations and predictability in the environment. They have a strong need to resist social norms and want to do things their own way. This may be oppositional but it also can be a means of expressing individuality and identity. When working to gain their cooperation, therapists need to be flexible and willing to negotiate while at the same time setting reasonable limits. When presented with musical instruments, a child might choose not to play in a conventional manner, for example, by tapping a tambourine with his hand, but instead wanting to play it with his feet. His desire might be accommodated by asking him to lie down, take off his shoes, and play with his bare feet so that he does not risk damaging the instrument. An added benefit might be that the sensitive soles of the feet provide a more intensive sensation, which many children seek out. When engaging in explorative musical play—whether singing or using instruments—there is room for children to use their ingenuity in finding unexpected and unique ways of expressing themselves.

INTERVENTIONS FOR CHILDREN WITH ASD

ASD has received increased attention in recent years as a result of an apparent dramatic rise in its incidence. ASD refers to a cluster of developmental disorders and includes a wide range, or spectrum, of symptoms, skills, and levels of disability (National Institute of Mental Health, 2016). People with ASD typically have difficulty communicating and interacting with others, they have limited interests, and they engage in repetitive behaviors as well as other behaviors that interfere with their ability to function socially.

Impairments in social–emotional reciprocity is one of the criteria for ASD (American Psychiatric Association, 2013). Difficulty in communicating effectively and making friends often leads to isolation and loneliness. Interspersing play activities, like music, movement, and singing, with more formal instruction or prompts to change behavior provides caregivers with a method for engaging children socially, creatively, and communicatively in a way that is appropriate for their developmental level (Berger, 2016; Macintyre, 2015). These activities offer children with habitual behavior patterns alternate, more fulfilling means of self-expression. Macintyre (2015) analyzed the ways in which experienced professionals work with children with ASD. When these ways were pooled, Macintyre found that these experts use strategies that involve building a warm and respectful rapport, establishing routines, encouraging play, and being positive. Macintyre also emphasized the importance of working with children's strengths and preferences. Tapping into the musical sensibilities of children with ASD can provide a bridge to their inner worlds and create a connection with the treatment provider.

Early intervention is recommended when considering treatment options for children with ASD, yet it can be difficult to determine what type of intervention will be most effective for a particular child. There has been considerable evidence showing that early intervention can be very helpful for children with ASD, with naturalistic developmental behavioral programs such as the Early Start Denver Model (ESDM) resulting in major gains in learning, communicating, and social skills (Rogers, Dawson, & Vismara, 2012; Rogers, Vivanti, & Rocha, 2017). Behavioral teaching and learning, as embodied in ABA, and stimulating emotional attachment through social interaction usually form the basis of early intervention (Fein, Helt, Brennan, & Barton, 2016) as well as later treatment.

Music can be a natural source of strength, communication, and ability for a child with ASD. There is a long history of using music therapeutically with children with autism (Alvin, 1978; Nordoff & Robbins, 2007). In 2015, music therapy was officially recognized by the National Autism Center as an "Emerging Intervention." As shown earlier, singing can stimulate neural pathways for language through rhythmic interpersonal exchange. Music can bypass cognitive processes and language to directly stimulate emotions and intensify emotional experiences. As a result, it can help children with ASD better understand and regulate their own emotions and learn to recognize emotions in others. Evidence suggests that individuals with ASD do not have difficulty recognizing simple emotions in music and may show an affinity for music and even superior abilities in processing some aspects of music (Molnar-Szakacs et al., 2009). Music therapists are specifically trained to pick up the vocal sounds, body movements, and activities of children who may seem remote and difficult to reach, and put them in a musical context that fosters communication (Brown, 1994).

Programs that incorporate behavioral, developmental, and naturalistic principles have shown how parents and other caregivers can use various strategies, including songs and music, to help children to communicate, improve social interactions, and increase play skills from an early age. Core skills such as imitation and joint attention can be learned through back-and-forth interchanges with sound. Parents can echo the sounds the child makes to convey that he has been heard and that his vocalizations are meaningful and important. They can also sing songs and highlight a "target" word or phrase by singing louder or slower. After singing the song for a few weeks, the child may try to put in the word himself, or make a sound in its place (Rogers et al., 2012, pp. 170–171). As shown earlier in this chapter, singing a song about a routine, such as breakfast, bath time, or going to sleep, can facilitate the transition and normalize the routine, as well as adding language and increasing communication. Some music therapists are integrating the behavioral focus of ABA-based programs with developmental goals and creating new models for parents and caregivers (Hernandez-Ruiz, 2018).

Therapists without specialized training can use music on a supportive level to stimulate awareness, communication, and participation. Some examples of how to become more aware of the child's experience of music are provided in the "Recommendations for Practice" section at the end of this chapter. The following example illustrates the powerful ways in which music can soothe and calm a distressed child, opening an opportunity for more intensive work.

VIGNETTE

I (J. C. B.) was working with Tyler, a 5-year-old child with severe receptive and expressive communication issues related to his diagnosis of ASD. His presenting issue, however, was his refusal to interact with other children. When at school, he would strike out whenever another child came too close to him and move away from the group during circle time. His teacher felt music might help him to gradually interact with another person and provide opportunities for healthy, situation-appropriate self-expression. Tyler immediately took to the music, playing instruments one after the other, yet not playing any one of them for very long. While he avoided direct contact with me, he seemed to be listening and responding to the piano music I played.

After just two sessions, Tyler began to reject the instruments and throw them forcefully across the room. These included metal horns and other small instruments that became dangerous projectiles in his hands. I felt I had no choice but to remove these instruments from the room, for his safety and mine. He threw chairs, so these also were removed. I thought the solution would be to bring in a large standing drum, which would be too heavy for him to move. But I was mistaken—if Tyler could not pick it up and throw it, he could still knock it over. This was taken out as well. That left just the piano and the piano bench, which I was sitting on. In the absence of any reason for Tyler's change in behavior, I wondered if his aggression was a defense against his feelings of burgeoning intimacy with me, which may have made him feel vulnerable and frightened. My immediate challenge was to deal with his behavior and find some positive way to interact with him. With the room emptied of its contents, and nothing left to fight against (except, perhaps, me, which he did not do), Tyler seemed to let go of his rage. He lay on the floor, his body calm, and began to vocalize in response to gentle piano playing and singing. I answered his sounds, in turn, and we had a musical conversation with our vocalizations that led to the beginning of a cooperative working relationship. In this case, music established a new pattern of interaction that was soothing and sustained. As a child acquires new skills through repeated positive experiences such as this, his sense of self expands, and he learns that he can approach other people and interact in satisfying ways. This brings him into closer contact with others and lessens his sense of isolation.

For Tyler, listening to music that was calming helped him achieve an internal state of stillness and tranquility. Music can serve as a natural analgesic in this way and assist children in reaching a state of integration and connectedness. Tyler's ability to vocalize and be part of the music indicated to me that he was capable of developing communication skills. Finding and using these types of alternative methods, that is, approaches that have minimal physiological and neurological side effects, are crucial to the treatment of children with ASD. Sometimes, music can have unexpected effects as well, as shown in the following example.

VIGNETTE

Timothy, age 2½, was diagnosed with ASD and presented with repetitive patterns of behavior, a lack of language development, and symptoms that included hand flapping and anxiety. In the first session, the therapist started to play the guitar and sing softly to him, and he fell into a deep sleep. The therapist tried to wake him, wanting to make the best use of his weekly half-hour. She sang to him, strummed the guitar loudly, even beat the drum with a hard mallet, but nothing roused him. This happened for the first three sessions. Realizing that her efforts to stimulate awareness and interaction were in vain, the therapist let him sleep and played soothing, peaceful music for him. She reluctantly approached Timothy's mother to tell her what was happening, concerned that she would view Timothy's sleeping as a lack of progress and withdraw him from therapy, but was surprised by her reaction. His mother was delighted that he was sleeping in his sessions—"This child never sleeps!" Apparently, the music relaxed him enough so that he could let go and allow himself to fall asleep. It is quite possible that even while he was sleeping, he was taking in the music on an unconscious level. Timothy soon moved out of his "sleeping" phase in therapy and became more active in his sessions.

SUMMARY

Children who have behavioral, emotional, and communication problems are often hard to treat, due to their tendency to reject contact and, sometimes, strike out. Compounding the difficulty in finding effective treatment options, many have comorbid issues. Given the extreme behaviors and dramatic emotional swings these children often experience, many practitioners use ABA and/or pharmacological behavior management, yet alternative treatments, including music, when integrated into treatment consistently, can have immediate and lasting effects on the child. The recommendations we provide can help you incorporate music and instrumental play into your work. A word of caution: music is a powerful medium and given the changeable nature of the children we discuss in this chapter, it is important to stay attuned to when it might be overwhelming or overstimulating. If you have even an inkling this might be happening, stop the music and redirect to another activity. We encourage you to review the following recommendations, work with them, and adapt some of the strategies to your own practice to the best of your abilities. Balancing the creative energy of music with structure and an ear to when limits need to be imposed offers a wonderful way for you to connect, play, and communicate with your young clients.

RECOMMENDATIONS FOR PRACTICE

As seen in this chapter, there are myriad ways music can be safely introduced into treatment of children who suffer from severe disorders. Being comfortable engaging in musical interactions is crucial to success, for a child with acute issues can often sense insecurity or anxiety in a therapist and try to capitalize on it. For this reason, we recommend you experiment with different ways to imagine what it is like for your client to experience the world and music.

- Find a quiet place to sit, with no disturbances to interrupt you.
  - Picture the child in your mind's eye: What does he look like? How does he move? What does he sound like? Hear his words and vocalizations and listen to them deeply: What is his emotional tone? What is he trying to communicate that his words or sounds do not say, but you can hear in his tone, rhythms, and pitches? What is the meaning behind his sounds?
  - Replicate his sounds with your own voice: What does it feel like? What is the internal sensation? Is it happy, anxious, or distressed?
  - While in this quiet place, take a few moments to again picture the child in your mind. How does he hear the world around him? How

do voices, words, traffic, television, etc., affect him? Is he able to make sense of these things?
- Now say his name. Repeat it several times. Imagine him responding to you stating his name.
- Next, sing his name. Does this sound or feel different from just saying his name? How do you think he would hear this? Sing it several times, experimenting with the emphases and rises or falls in melody. Become comfortable singing his name.

Strategies Described in Prior Chapters That Are Adaptable to Working with Children with Severe Disorders

- Sing a song known to the child (e.g., "Ring Around the Rosy" with Autumn), and be creative in acting it out ("We all fall down") and changing the words ("We all fly away").
- Substitute lyrics to a familiar song. Try writing one verse to past self, one verse to present self, and one verse to future self.
- Use vowel or "la" sounds when singing familiar songs; focusing on melody without words accesses a preverbal area of the brain, making it easier for a child with language difficulties to engage with you.
- Listen to carefully selected music together. Songs should have a clear structure of chorus and verses, while other forms of music that do not have words, for example, classical music, need to be appealing to children and not have heavy overlays of emotion or dissonance.
- Use a playful, unpressured approach to involve children in vocalizing or instrumental play; sing about a cat or dog, or about the car the child travels in.
- Use props such as scarves or stretch bands and move to music.

Group Turn Taking

- Seat the children in chairs in a tight circle.
- Choose two songs familiar to the children; these can be from popular genres or we also recommend choosing songs that their parents or caregivers prefer. If the therapist has music skills, play a simple two-chord progression. Varying it in terms of tempo and dynamics will effectively contain the activity.

- Have one small percussion instrument ready to pass around the circle; a maraca, egg shaker, or small hand drum work well for this exercise.
- Explain the rules of the game to the children: when the music starts, the child who holds the instrument starts playing it, and when the music stops (at the discretion of the therapist) the child stops playing and hands the instrument to the person to his left. There is no talking or physical contact (other than passing the instrument) during the game.
- Model how to do this once, then begin.
- Once the circle has been completed, repeat with a different instrument, stop the activity and review how it went, or move on to another activity.

Offering Choices

- In individual therapy, ask your client if he prefers a slow or fast song and play a recording that fits his choice.
    - Client and therapist choose an instrument.
    - Both therapist and client play instruments to accompany the music.
- Play a "Name Game":
    - Introduce the activity as a fun way to say your name.
    - State name verbally as it is usually said.
    - Ask your client if he would like to say his name fast or slow, loud or soft.
    - Both therapist and child say/chant the name in the way chosen.
    - Expand on this by introducing more choices such as starting soft and getting louder, holding some syllables longer than others.

Additional Considerations When Working with This Population

- Maintain a high awareness of boundaries, physical space, and safety.
- Have a heightened awareness of when to stop if a musical intervention is not having a positive result; sensory overload can happen quickly when engaged in music activities.
- Have a back-up plan. Children's responses can quickly change, so be prepared to shift gears when needed.

- Know the limits of what you can do and when to make a referral to a music or developmental disabilities therapist.
- When working in a hospital or institutional setting, be mindful of the noise level on the unit. It is important to be aware of the sensory sensitivities of your client and of the other children.
- Try a multimodal approach, incorporating movement or art based on the child's needs and interests.
- Collaborate with other therapists, especially with other creative arts therapists.

Postscript

> The final paradox of music, perhaps, is that it is through our universal musical humanness that the uniqueness of each of us as an individual can be so fully celebrated.
> —Brown (1994, p. 24)

In closing, we are reminded of Clive Robbins's articulation of what he called "the goodbye effect." When using music in a therapeutic way, children respond in unexpected and sometimes surprising ways. There are times, however, when children resist music and resist the urge to engage and participate. We have both experienced times when we start to sing or play a goodbye song as a way of marking the end of the session, and suddenly a child will begin to play, or move, or sing.

Sarah, a clinical psychologist who uses music in her practice, relayed this story: Roger was a 12-year-old boy with anger issues who, for the first session, would not respond to verbal questions and ignored Sarah's attempts to engage him in musical play. After 10 minutes of probing and offering music, Sarah sat with Roger for several minutes in silence. She then picked up a small hand drum and began to play a steady beat as she chanted, "It's time to say goodbye, it's time to say goodbye, we'll see each other again." She did not look at Roger as she did this, but saw out of the corner of her eye as he picked up his head, looked around the room, and reached out to the tall floor tubano drum she had placed in front of him earlier in the session. He began to lightly tap the drum, mirroring her steady beat. Sarah stopped chanting and continued to drum, letting him stop when he wanted to. After a couple of minutes of playing together, Roger stopped and stood up. Sarah ceased playing immediately and, as they walked out together, thanked him for coming. Roger replied, "Okay, see you next week."

Initiating a goodbye can unlock a wave of expression and involvement. We hope that here, at the conclusion of this book, you experience a similar phenomenon, and will have ideas for how to bring music into the therapy room and that the ideas and suggestions we have presented are like seeds that will continue to germinate and bring new growth to your work.

References

Afolabi, O. E. (2015). Domestic violence, risky family environment and children: A bio-psychology perspective. *International Journal of Special Education, 30*(2), 44–56.

Aigen, K. (2014). Music-centered dimensions of Nordoff–Robbins music therapy. *Music Therapy Perspectives, 32*(1), 18–29.

Ainsworth, M. D. S. (1967). *Infancy in Uganda: Infant care and the growth of love.* Baltimore: Johns Hopkins University Press.

Ainsworth, M. D. S. (1979). Infant–mother attachment. *American Psychologist, 34*(10), 932–937.

Ainsworth, M. D. S., Blehar, M. C., Waters, E., & Wall, S. (1978). *Patterns of attachment: A psychological study of the Strange Situation.* Mahwah, NJ: Erlbaum.

Allen, J. P., & Tan, J. S. (2016). The multiple facets of attachment in adolescence. In J. Cassidy & P. R. Shaver (Eds.), *Handbook of attachment: Theory, research, and clinical applications* (3rd ed., pp. 399–415). New York: Guilford Press.

Alvin, J. (1978). *Music therapy for the autistic child.* London: Oxford University Press.

American Academy of Child and Adolescent Psychiatry. (2009). Child and adolescent mental illness statistics. Retrieved from *www.aacap.org/aacap/ families_and_youth/Family_Resources/Child_and_Adolescent_Mental_ Illness_and_Drug_Abuse_Statistics.aspx.*

American Psychiatric Association. (2013). *Diagnostic and statistical manual of mental disorders* (5th ed.). Arlington, VA: Author.

Arlen, H., & Harburg, Y. (1939). *Somewhere over the rainbow.* New York: WinStar Home Entertainment.

Austin, D. S. (2002). The voice of trauma: A wounded healer's perspective. In J. P. Sutton (Ed.), *Music, music therapy and trauma: International perspectives* (pp. 231–259). London: Jessica Kingsley.

Austin, D. S., & Dvorkin, J. (1998). Resistance in individual music therapy. In K. E. Bruscia (Ed.), *The dynamics of music psychotherapy* (pp. 121–135). Gilsum, NH: Barcelona.

Baron, S. (2014, June). Ending the therapeutic silent treatment. *Play Therapy*, pp. 6–9.

Bartholomew, J. B., Jowers, E. M., Errisuriz, V. L., Vaughn, S., & Roberts, G. (2017). A cluster randomized control trial to assess the impact of active learning on child activity, attention control, and academic outcomes: The Texas I-CAN Trial. *Contemporary Clinical Trials, 1*, 81–86.

Beck, L., D'Antonio, N., & Lyon, L. (2014). Why internationally adopted children are at risk for RAD. Retrieved from www.attach-china.org/whyinternational.html.

Bedoin, N., Brisseau, L., Molinier, P., Roch, D., & Tillmann, B. (2016). Temporally regular musical primes facilitate subsequent syntax processing in children with specific language impairment. *Frontiers in Neuroscience, 10*(245), 1–11.

Beer, L. E. (2011). A model for clinical decision-making in music therapy: Planning and implementing improvisational experiences. *Music Therapy Perspectives, 29*(2), 117–125.

Beer, L. E. (2017). The role of the music therapist in training caregivers of people who have advanced dementia. *Nordic Journal of Music Therapy, 26*(2), 185–199.

Beer, L. E., & Lee, K. V. (2017). Music therapy and procedural support: Opportunities for practice. *Music and Medicine, 9*(4), 262–268.

Berger, D. S. (2016). *Kids, music 'n' autism: Bringing out the music in your child*. London: Jessica Kingsley.

Berkowitz, A. L. (2016). The cognitive neuroscience of improvisation. In G. E. Lewis & B. Piekut (Eds.), *The Oxford handbook of critical improvisation studies* (Vol. 1, pp. 56–73). New York: Oxford University Press.

Berlin, L. J., Zeanah, C. H., & Lieberman, A. F. (2016). Prevention and intervention programs to support early attachment security: A move to the level of the community. In J. Cassidy & P. R. Shaver (Eds.), *Handbook of attachment: Theory, research, and clinical applications* (3rd ed., pp. 739–758). New York: Guilford Press.

Berlin, L. J., Ziv, Y., Amaya-Jackson, L., & Greenberg, M. T. (2005). *Enhancing early attachments*. New York: Guilford Press.

Bieleninik, L., Ghetti, C., & Gold, C. (2016). Music therapy for preterm infants and their parents: A meta-analysis. *Pediatrics, 138*(3), e20160971.

Birnbaum, J. C. (2013). *Healing childhood trauma through music and play*. Gilsum, NH: Barcelona.

Borczon, R. M. (2015). Music therapy for survivors of traumatic events. In B. L. Wheeler (Ed.), *Music therapy handbook* (pp. 390–400). New York: Guilford Press.

Bowlby, J. (1982). *Attachment and loss: Vol. 1. Attachment.* London: Hogarth Press.

Bowlby, J. (2005). *The making and breaking of affectional bonds.* New York: Routledge Classics. (Original work published 1979)

Bratton, S. C., & Swan, A. (2017). Status of play therapy research. In R. L. Steen (Ed.), *Emerging research in play therapy, child counseling, and consultation* (pp. 1–19). Hershey, PA: IGI Global.

Brief, A., & Motowidlo, S. (1986). Pro social organizational behaviors. *Academy of Management Review, 11*(4), 710–725.

Briere, J. N., & Scott, C. (2014). *Principles of trauma therapy: A guide to symptoms, evaluation, and treatment* (DSM-5 update). Thousand Oaks, CA: Sage.

Briggs, C. A. (1991). A model for understanding musical development. *Music Therapy 10*(1), 1–21.

Briggs, C. A. (2015). Developmental approaches. In B. L. Wheeler (Ed.), *Music therapy handbook* (pp. 172–182). New York: Guilford Press.

Briggs, C. A. & Bruscia, K. (1985, November). *Developmental models for understanding musical development.* Paper presented at the Joint Conference on the Creative Arts Therapies, National Coalition of Arts Therapy Associations, New York.

Bromberg, P. M. (2006). *Awakening the dreamer: Clinical journeys.* Mahwah, NJ: Analytic Press.

Brown, L. S. (2017). The influence of music on facial emotion recognition in children with autism spectrum disorder and neurotypical children. *Journal of Music Therapy, 54*(1), 55–79.

Brown, M. W. (2007). *Goodnight moon.* New York: HarperCollins.

Brown, S. M. K. (1994). Autism and music therapy: Is change possible, and why music? *Journal of British Music Therapy, 8*(1), 15–25.

Calikusu Incekar, M., & Balci, S. (2017). The effect of training on noise reduction in neonatal intensive care units. *Journal for Specialists in Pediatric Nursing, 22*(3), e12181.

Carey, L. (2006). Introduction. In L. Carey (Ed.), *Expressive and creative arts methods for trauma survivors* (pp. 15–20). Philadelphia: Jessica Kingsley.

Carpentier, S. M., Moreno, S., & McIntosh, A. R. (2016). Short-term music training enhances complex, distributed neural communication during music and linguistic tasks. *Journal of Cognitive Neuroscience, 29*(10), 1603–1612.

Cassidy, J., & Shaver, P. R. (Eds.). (2016). *Handbook of attachment: Theory, research, and clinical applications* (3rd ed.). New York: Guilford Press.

Cavanagh, M., Quinn, D., Duncan, D., Graham, T., & Balbuena, L. (2017).

Oppositional defiant disorder is better conceptualized as a disorder of emotional regulation. *Journal of Attention Disorders, 21*(5), 381–389.

Chau, C. J., & Horner, A. (2015). The effects of pitch and dynamics on the emotional characteristics of piano sounds. In *Proceedings of the 42nd International Computer Music Conference*. Denton, TX: Center for Experimental Music, University of North Texas.

Chen-Hafteck, L., & Mang, E. (2018). Music and language in early childhood development and learning. In G. E. McPherson & G. E. Welch (Eds.), *Music learning and teaching in infancy, childhood, and adolescence: An Oxford handbook of music education* (Vol. 2, pp. 40–57). New York: Oxford University Press.

Cheung, M. C., Chan, A. S., Liu, Y., Law, D., & Wong, C. W. (2017). Music training is associated with cortical synchronization reflected in EEG coherence during verbal memory encoding. *PLOS ONE, 12*(3), e0174906.

Cohen, J. A., Mannarino, A. P., & Deblinger, E. (2017). *Treating trauma and traumatic grief in children and adolescents* (2nd ed.). New York: Guilford Press.

Cohen, J. A., Mannarino, A. P., & Knudsen, K. (2004). Treating childhood traumatic grief: A pilot study. *Journal of the American Academy of Child and Adolescent Psychiatry, 43*(10), 1225–1233.

Collins, F. S., & Fleming, R. (2017). Sound health: An NIH–Kennedy Center initiative to explore music and the mind. *JAMA, 317*(24), 2470–2471.

Compton, S. N., Peris, T. S., Almirall, D., Birmaher, B., Sherrill, J., Kendall, P. C., . . . Albano, A. M. (2014). Predictors and moderators of treatment response in childhood anxiety disorders: Results from the CAMS trial. *Journal of Consulting and Clinical Psychology, 82*(2), 212–224.

Condon, W. S., & Sander, L. W. (1974). Synchrony demonstrated between movements of the neonate and adult speech. *Child Development, 45*, 456–462.

Corbeil, M., Trehub, S. E., & Peretz, I. (2016). Singing delays the onset of infant distress. *Infancy, 21*(3), 373–391.

Cornacchio, D., Bry, L. J., Sanchez, A. L., Poznanski, B., & Comer, J. S. (2017). Psychosocial treatment and prevention of conduct problems in early childhood. In J. E. Lochman & W. Matthys (Eds.), *The Wiley handbook of disruptive and impulse-control disorders* (pp. 443–449). Chichester, UK: Wiley.

Crenshaw, D. A. (2006). *Evocative strategies in child and adolescent psychotherapy*. New York: Jason Aronson.

Crenshaw, D. A. (2017). Resistance in child psychotherapy: Playing hide-and-seek. In C. A. Malchiodi & D. A. Crenshaw (Eds.), *What to do when children clam up in psychotherapy* (pp. 18–37). New York: Guilford Press.

Crenshaw, D. A., Brooks, R., & Goldstein, S. (2015). *Play therapy interventions to enhance resilience*. New York: Guilford Press.

Csikszentmihalyi, M. (1990). *Flow: The psychology of optimal experience*. New York: Harper Collins.

Davies, A., Barwick, N., & Richards, E. (2015). *Group music therapy: A group analytic approach*. New York: Routledge.

Davis, K. M. (2010). Music and the expressive arts with children experiencing trauma. *Journal of Creativity in Mental Health, 5*, 125–133.

Davis, W., & Hadley, S. (2015). A history of music therapy. In B. L. Wheeler (Ed.), *Music therapy handbook* (pp. 17–28). New York: Guilford Press.

DeCasper, A. J., & Fifer, W. P. (1980). Of human bonding: Newborns prefer their mothers' voices. *Science, 208*, 1174–1176.

DeKlyen, M., & Greenberg, M. T. (2016). Attachment and psychopathology in childhood. In J. Cassidy & P. R. Shaver (Eds.), *Handbook of attachment: Theory, research, and clinical applications* (3rd ed., pp. 639–666). New York: Guilford Press.

DeRobertis, E. M. (2008). *Humanizing child development theory: A holistic approach*. New York: iUniverse.

Dimeff, L., & Linehan, M. M. (2001). Dialectical behavior therapy in a nutshell. *California Psychologist, 34*(3), 10–13.

Duarte, A. (2017). Getting together, playing together, healing together. In S. Hart (Ed.), *Inclusion, play and empathy: Neuroaffective development in children's groups* (pp. 250–265). Philadelphia: Jessica Kingsley.

Eisenberg, N., Spinrad, T. L., & Valiente, C. (2016). Emotion-related self-regulation, and children's social, psychological, and academic functioning. In C. Balter & C. S. Tamis-LeMonda (Eds.), *Child psychology: A handbook of contemporary issues* (3rd ed., pp. 219–244). New York: Routledge.

Elvers, P., Fischinger, T., & Steffens, J. (2018, June). Music listening as self-enhancement: Effects of empowering music on momentary explicit and implicit self-esteem. *Psychology of Music, 46*(3), 307–325.

Fein, D., Helt, M., Brennan, L., & Barton, M. (2016). *The activity kit for babies and toddlers at risk: How to use everyday routines to build social and communication skills*. New York: Guilford Press.

Fogg-Rogers, L., Buetow, S., Talmage, A., McCann, C. M., Leão, S. H., Tippett, L., . . . Purdy, S. C. (2016). Choral singing therapy following stroke or Parkinson's disease: An exploration of participants' experiences. *Disability and Rehabilitation, 38*(10), 952–962.

Ford, J. D. (2017). Treatment implications of altered affect regulation and information processing following child maltreatment. *Psychiatric Annals, 35*(5), 410–419.

Galewitz, H. (2001). *Music: A book of quotations*. N. Chelmsford, MA: Courier.

Garrido, S. (2009). Rumination and sad music: A review of the literature and a future direction. In *Proceedings of the 2nd International Conference on Music Communication Science*, Sydney, Australia.

Gaskill, R. L., & Perry, B. D. (2014). The neurobiological power of play: Using the neurosequential model of therapeutics to guide play in the healing process. In C. A. Malchiodi & D. A. Crenshaw (Eds.), *Creative arts and play therapy for attachment problems* (pp. 178–194). New York: Guilford Press.

Gaston, E. T. (1968). *Music in therapy.* New York: Macmillan.

Gazzaniga, M. S. (2018). *Psychological science* (6th ed.). New York: Norton.

Gil, E. (2015). Posttraumatic play: A robust path to resilience. In D. A. Crenshaw, R. Brooks, & S. Goldstein (Eds.), *Play therapy interventions to enhance resilience* (pp. 107–125). New York: Guilford Press.

Gil, E. (2017). *Posttraumatic play in children: What clinicians need to know.* New York: Guilford Press.

Glen, N. L. (2017). Why do we "Skip to My Lou," anyway?: Teaching play party songs in historical context. *General Music Today, 30*(2), 4–10.

Goldstein, B., & Ogden, P. (2017). Playing with possibilities: Sensorimotor psychotherapy with younger clients in individual, family, and group psychotherapy. In S. Hart (Ed.), *Inclusion, play and empathy: Neuroaffective development in children's groups* (pp. 228–248). Philadelphia: Jessica Kingsley.

Grau-Sánchez, J., Ramos, N., Duarte, E., Särkämö, T., & Rodríguez-Fornells, A. (2017, April). Time course of motor gains induced by music-supported therapy after stroke: An exploratory case study. *Neuropsychology,* pp. 1–13.

Greene, R. W., & Ablon, J. S. (2006). *Treating explosive kids: The collaborative problem-solving approach.* New York: Guilford Press.

Guilmartin, K. K., & Levinowitz, L. M. (2008). *Introducing music together.* Princeton, NJ: Music Together.

Guralnick, M. J. (2017). Early intervention for children with intellectual disabilities: An update. *Journal of Applied Research in Intellectual Disabilities, 30*(2), 211–229.

Hadiwijaya, H., Klimstra, T. A., Vermunt, J. K., Branje, S. J., & Meeus, W. H. (2017). On the development of harmony, turbulence, and independence in parent–adolescent relationships: A five-wave longitudinal study. *Journal of Youth and Adolescence, 46*(8), 1772–1788.

Hallam, S. (2016, June). The impact of actively making music on the intellectual, social and personal development of children and young people: A summary. *Voices: A World Forum for Music Therapy, 16*(2).

Hart, S. (2017). Empathy and compassion are acquired skills. In S. Hart (Ed.), *Inclusion, play and empathy: Neuroaffective development in children's groups* (pp. 55–78). Philadelphia: Jessica Kingsley.

Harvey, A. (2017). *Music, evolution, and the harmony of souls.* Oxford, UK: Oxford University Press.

Heidegger, M. (1995). *The fundamental concepts of metaphysics: World, finitude, solitude.* Bloomington, IN: Indiana University Press.

Hernandez-Ruiz, E. (2018). Music therapy and Early Start Denver Model to teach social communication strategies to parents of preschoolers with ASD: A feasibility study. *Music Therapy Perspectives, 36*(1), 26–39.

Hetland, L., & Winner, E. (2004). Cognitive transfer from arts education to non-arts outcomes: Research evidence and policy implications. In E. Eisner & M. Day (Eds.), *Handbook of research and policy in art education* (pp. 135–162). Mahwah, NJ: Erlbaum.

Hodges, D. A., & Sebald, D. C. (2011). *Music in the human experience.* New York: Routledge.

Holck, U., & Jacobsen, S. L. (2017). Inclusion, children's groups, music therapy. In S. Hart (Ed.), *Inclusion, play and empathy: Neuroaffective development in children's groups* (pp. 159–180). Philadelphia: Jessica Kingsley.

Hughes, D. (2014). Attachment-focused therapeutic interventions. In P. Holmes & S. Farnfield (Eds.), *The Routledge handbook of attachment: Implications and interventions* (pp. 104–116). New York: Routledge.

Ilie, G., & Thompson, W. F. (2006). A comparison of acoustic cues in music and speech for three dimensions of affect. *Music Perception: An Interdisciplinary Journal, 23*(4), 319–330.

Isenberg, C. (2015). Psychodynamic approaches. In B. L. Wheeler (Ed.), *Music therapy handbook* (pp. 133–147). New York: Guilford Press.

Jalongo, M. R., & Collins, M. (1985). Singing with young children!: Folk singing for nonmusicians. *Young Children, 40*(2), 17–22.

Javdani, S., Sadeh, N., Donenberg, G. R., Emerson, E. M., Houck, C., & Brown, L. K. (2017). Affect recognition among adolescents in therapeutic schools: Relationships with posttraumatic stress disorder and conduct disorder symptoms. *Child and Adolescent Mental Health, 22*(1), 42–48.

Karmonik, C., Brandt, A., Anderson, J. R., Brooks, F., Lytle, J., Silverman, E., & Frazier, J. T. (2016). Music listening modulates functional connectivity and information flow in the human brain. *Brain Connectivity, 6*(8), 632–641.

Kawakami, A., Furukawa, K., Katahira, K., & Okanoya, K. (2013). Sad music induces pleasant emotion. *Frontiers in Psychology, 4*(311), 1–15.

Kinniburgh, K. J., Blaustein, M., Spinazzola, J., & van der Kolk, B. A. (2017). Attachment, self-regulation, and competency: A comprehensive intervention framework for children with complex trauma. *Psychiatric Annals, 35*(5), 424–430.

Knight, S., Spiro, N., & Cross, I. (2017). Look, listen and learn: Exploring effects of passive entrainment on social judgements of observed others. *Psychology of Music, 45*(1), 99–115.

Ko, E., Seidl, A., Cristia, A., Reimchen, M., & Soderstrom, M. (2016). Entrainment of prosody in the interaction of mothers with their young children. *Journal of Child Language, 43*(2), 284–309.

Koelsch, S. (2009). A neuroscientific perspective on music therapy. *Annals of the New York Academy of Sciences, 1169*(1), 374–384.

Koelsch, S. (2012). *Brain and music.* Hoboken, NJ: Wiley-Blackwell.

Kossak, M. S. (2009). Therapeutic attunement: A transpersonal view of expressive arts therapy. *Arts in Psychotherapy, 36*(1), 13–18.

Kottman, T. (2001). *Play therapy: Basics and beyond*. Alexandria, VA: American Counseling Association.

Kramer, D. N., & Landolt, M. A. (2011). Characteristics and efficacy of early psychological interventions in children and adolescents after single trauma: A meta-analysis. *European Journal of Psychotraumatology, 2*(1), 7858. Retrieved from *www.tandfonline.com/doi/pdf/10.3402/ejpt.v2i0.7858?needAccess=true*.

Kraus, N., & Chandrasekaran, B. (2010). Music training for the development of auditory skills. *Neuroscience, 11*(8), 599–604.

Kraus, N., Hornickel, J., Strait, D. L., Slater, J., & Thompson, E. (2014). Engagement in community music classes sparks neuroplasticity and language development in children from disadvantaged backgrounds. *Frontiers in Psychology, 5*(1403), 1–9.

Langdon, G. S. (2015). Music therapy for adults with mental illness. In B. L. Wheeler (Ed.), *Music therapy handbook* (pp. 341–353). New York: Guilford Press.

Levine, P. A., & Frederick, A. (1997). *Waking the tiger: Healing trauma: The innate capacity to transform overwhelming experiences*. Berkeley, CA: North Atlantic Books.

Levinge, A. (2015). *The music of being: Music therapy, Winnicott and the school of object relations*. Philadelphia: Jessica Kingsley.

Levitin, D. J. (2007). *This is your brain on music: The science of a human obsession*. New York: Plume Penguin.

Levitin, D. J., Grahn, J., & London, J. (2018). The psychology of music: Rhythm and movement. *Annual Review of Psychology, 69*(1), 51–75.

Lieberman, A. F., & Van Horn, P. (2008). *Psychotherapy with infants and young children: Repairing the effects of stress and trauma on early attachment*. New York: Guilford Press.

Loewy, J. (2007). *Music therapy in the NICU* (2nd ed.). New York: Louis & Lucille Armstrong Music Therapy Program, Beth Israel Medical Center.

Loewy, J. (2015). NICU music therapy: Song of kin as critical lullaby in research and practice. *Annals of the New York Academy of Sciences, 1337*(1), 178–185.

Loewy, J., Stewart, K., Dassler, A.-M., Telsey, A., & Homel, P. (2013). The effects of music therapy on vital signs, feeding, and sleep in premature infants. *Pediatrics, 131*(5), 902–918.

Lonie, D. (2010). *Early years evidence review: Assessing the outcomes of early years music making*. London: Youth Music.

Lorenzo, O., Herrera, L., Hernandez-Candelas, M., & Badea, M. (2014). Influence of music training on language development. A longitudinal study. *Procedia—Social and Behavioral Sciences, 128*, 527–530.

Loumeau-May, L. V., Seibel-Nicol, E., Hamilton, M. P., & Malchiodi, C. A. (2015). Art therapy as an intervention for mass terrorism and violence. In C. A. Malchiodi (Ed.), *Creative interventions with traumatized children* (2nd ed., pp. 94–125). New York: Guilford Press.

Loxton, N. J., Mitchell, R., Dingle, G. A., & Sharman, L. S. (2016). How to tame your BAS: Reward sensitivity and music involvement. *Personality and Individual Differences, 97*, 35–39.

Lyon, L. (2005). Children's reactions to trauma. Retrieved from www.attach-china.org/children'sreacti.html.

Lyon, L., D'Antonio, N., & Beck, L. (2014). Complex trauma in post-institutionalized children. Retrieved from www.attach-china.org/traumainpost-ins.html.

Macintyre, C. (2015). *Strategies to support children with autism and other complex needs: Resources for teachers, support staff and parents*. New York: Routledge.

Malchiodi, C. A. (1998). *Understanding children's drawings*. New York: Guilford Press.

Malchiodi, C. A. (2015). Calm, connection, and confidence: Using art therapy to enhance resilience in traumatized children. In D. A. Crenshaw, R. Brooks, & S. Goldstein (Eds.), *Play therapy interventions to enhance resilience* (pp. 126–145). New York: Guilford Press.

Malchiodi, C. A., & Crenshaw, D. A. (Eds.). (2017). *What to do when children clam up in psychotherapy*. New York: Guilford Press.

Maslow, A. (1964). *Religions, values and peak experiences*. New York: Viking Press.

McKay, D., Abramowitz, J. S., & Storch, E. A. (2017). Obsessive–compulsive and related disorders: Where have we been? In J. S. Abramowitz, D. McKay, & E. A. Storch, (Eds.), *The Wiley handbook of obsessive–compulsive disorders* (Vol. 1, pp. 1–5). New York: Wiley.

McLeod, B. D., Sutherland, K. S., Martinez, R. G., Conroy, M. A., Snyder, P. A., & Southam-Gerow, M. A. (2017). Identifying common practice elements to improve social, emotional, and behavioral outcomes of young children in early childhood classrooms. *Prevention Science, 18*(2), 204–213.

Mehrabian, A. (2017). Nonverbal communication. New York: Routledge.

Mitchell, S. A. (1988). *Relational concepts in psychoanalysis: An integration*. Cambridge, MA: Harvard University Press.

Molnar-Szakacs, I., Wang, M. J., Laugeson, E. A., Overy, K., Wu, W.-L., & Piggot, J. (2009). Autism, emotion recognition and the mirror neuron system: The case of music. *McGill Journal of Medicine, 12*(2), 87–98.

Mondonaro, J. (2016). Multiculturally focused medical music psychotherapy in affirming identity to facilitate optimal coping during hospitalization. *Music Therapy Perspectives, 34*(2), 154–160.

Morano, S., Ruiz, S., Hwang, J., Wertalki, J. L., Moeller, J., Karal, M. A., & Mulloy, A. (2017). Meta-analysis of single-case treatment effects on self-injurious behavior for individuals with autism and intellectual disabilities. *Autism and Developmental Language Impairments, 2*, 1–26.

Morata, T. C. (2007). Young people: Their noise and music exposures and the risk of hearing loss. *International Journal of Audiology, 46*(3), 111–112.

Moreno, S. (2009). Can music influence language and cognition? *Contemporary Music Review, 28*(3), 329–345.

Moreno, S., Bialystok, E., Barac, R., Schellenberg, E. G., Cepeda, N. J., & Chau, T. (2011). Short-term music training enhances verbal intelligence and executive function. *Psychological Science, 22*(11), 1425–1433.

Moreno, S., Marques, C., Santos, S., Santos M., Castro, S. L., & Besson, M. (2009). Musical training influences linguistic abilities in 8-year-old children: More evidence for brain plasticity. *Cerebral Cortex, 19*(3), 712–723.

National Autism Center. (2015). *Findings and conclusions: National Standards Project, Phase 2.* Randolph, MA: Author.

National Child Traumatic Stress Network. (n.d.-a). Psychological first aid. Retrieved from *www.nctsn.org/content/psychological-first-aid*.

National Child Traumatic Stress Network. (n.d.-b). Medical events and traumatic stress in children and families. Retrieved from *www.nctsn.org/nctsn_assets/pdfs/edu_materials/MedicalTraumaticStress.pdf*.

National Institute of Mental Health. (2016). Autism spectrum disorder. Retrieved from *www.nimh.nih.gov/health/topics/autism-spectrum-disorders-asd/index.shtml*.

Nielsen, J. A., Zielinski, B. A., Ferguson, M. A., Lainhart, J. E., & Anderson, J. S. (2013). An evaluation of the left-brain vs. right-brain hypothesis with resting state functional connectivity magnetic resonance imaging. *PLOS ONE, 8*(8), e71275.

Nietzsche, F. (1990). *Twilight of the idols.* New York: Penguin Books. (Original work published 1889)

Nordoff, P., & Robbins, C. (1961). *Pif-paf-poltrie.* Bryn Mawr, PA: Theodore Presser.

Nordoff, P., & Robbins, C. (1985). *Therapy in music for handicapped children.* London: Gollancz.

Nordoff, P., & Robbins, C. (2007). *Creative music therapy: A guide to fostering clinical musicianship* (2nd ed.). Gilsum, NH: Barcelona. (Original work published 1977)

Ogden, P., & Fisher, J. (2015). *Sensorimotor psychotherapy: Interventions for trauma and attachment.* New York: Norton.

Page, N. (1995). *Music as a way of knowing.* York, ME: Stenhouse.

Passanisi, A., Di Nuovo, S., Urgese, L., & Pirrone, C. (2015). The influence of musical expression on creativity and interpersonal relationships in children. *Procedia—Social and Behavioral Sciences, 191,* 2476–2480.

Patel, A. D. (2008). *Music, language and the brain.* New York: Oxford University Press.

Patel, A. D. (2017). Using music to study the evolution of cognitive mechanisms relevant to language. *Psychonomic Bulletin and Review, 24*(1), 177–180.

Patel, A. D., & Morgan, E. (2017). Exploring cognitive relations between prediction in language and music. *Cognitive Science, 41*(Suppl. 2), 303–320.

Pearce, C. (2016). *Short introduction to attachment and attachment disorder* (2nd ed.). London: Jessica Kingsley.
Perry, B. D. (2008). Foreword. In C. A. Malchiodi (Ed.), *Creative interventions with traumatized children* (pp. ix–xi). New York: Guilford Press.
Perry, B. D., & Szalavitz, M. (2006). *The boy who was raised as a dog*. New York: Basic Books.
Pickering, M. J., & Garrod, S. 2004. Toward a mechanistic psychology of dialogue. *Behavioral and Brain Sciences, 27*(2), 169–190.
Plamper, J. (2015). *The history of emotions: An introduction*. Oxford, UK: Oxford University Press.
Pliszka, S. R. (2015). Comorbid psychiatric disorders in children with ADHD. In R. A. Barkley (Ed.), *Attention-deficit hyperactivity disorder: A handbook for diagnosis and treatment* (pp. 140–168). New York: Guilford Press.
Porges, S. W. (2009). The polyvagal theory: New insights into adaptive reactions of the autonomic nervous system. *Cleveland Clinic Journal of Medicine, 76*(Suppl. 2), S86–S90.
Porges, S. W. (2010). Music therapy and trauma: Insights from the polyvagal theory. In K. Stewart (Ed.), *Music therapy and trauma: Bridging theory and clinical practice* (pp. 3–15). New York: Satchnote Press
Porges, S. W. (2011). *The polyvagal theory: Neurophysiological foundations of emotions, attachment, communication, and self-regulation*. New York: Norton.
Powell, B., Cooper, G., Hoffman, K., & Marvin, B. (2014). *The Circle of Security intervention: Enhancing attachment in early parent–child relationships*. New York: Guilford Press.
Powers, A., Etkin, A., Gyurak, A., Bradley, B., & Jovanovic, T. (2015). Associations between childhood abuse, posttraumatic stress disorder, and implicit emotion regulation deficits: Evidence from a low-income, inner-city population. *Psychiatry, 78*(3), 251–264.
Quinn, S. M., & Knoerlein, K. (2016). Developmental care and optimizing neurodevelopmental outcomes in the preterm and critically ill infant. In S. Bellini & M. J. Beaulieu (Eds.), *Neonatal advanced practice nursing: A case-based learning approach* (pp. 413–448). New York: Springer.
Rabinowitch, T. C., Cross, I., & Burnard, P. (2013). Long-term musical group interaction has a positive influence on empathy in children. *Psychology of Music, 41*(4), 484–498.
Ramsauer, B., Lotzin, A., Mühlhan, C., Romer, G., Nolte, T., Fonagy, P., & Powell, B. (2014). A randomized controlled trial comparing Circle of Security intervention and treatment as usual as interventions to increase attachment security in infants of mentally ill mothers: Study protocol. *BMC Psychiatry, 14*(1), 1–11.
Rauscher, F., Shaw, G., Levein, L., Wright, E., Dennis, W., & Newcomb, R. (1997). Music training causes long-term enhancement of preschool children's spatial–temporal reasoning. *Neurological Research, 19*(1), 2–8.

Robarts, J. Z. (2003). The healing function of improvised songs in music therapy with a child survivor of early trauma and sexual abuse. In S. Hadley (Ed.), *Psychodynamic music therapy: Case studies* (pp. 141–182). Gilsum, NH: Barcelona.

Robarts, J. Z. (2014). Music therapy with children with developmental trauma disorder. In C. A. Malchiodi & D. A. Crenshaw (Eds.), *Creative arts and play therapy for attachment problems* (pp. 67–83). New York: Guilford Press.

Robarts, J. Z. (2016). The remembered scream: Integrative music therapy with children with developmental trauma disorder. *Nordic Journal of Music Therapy, 25*(1), 63.

Robbins, C. (2005). *A journey into creative music therapy* (Vol. 3). Gilsum, NH: Barcelona.

Robbins, C., & Forinash, M. (1991). A time paradigm: Time as a multilevel phenomenon in music therapy. *Music Therapy, 10*(1), 46–57.

Rogenmoser, L., Kernbach, J., Schlaug, G., & Gaser, C. (2018). Keeping brains young with making music. *Brain Structure and Function, 223*(1), 1–9.

Rogers, S. J., Dawson, G., & Vismara, L. A. (2012). *An Early Start for your child with autism.* New York: Guilford Press.

Rogers, S. J., Vivanti, G., & Rocha, M. (2017). Helping young children with autism spectrum disorder develop social ability: The Early Start Denver Model approach. In J. B. Leaf (Ed.), *Handbook of social skills and autism spectrum disorder* (pp. 197–222). Cham, Switzerland: Springer.

Rossetti, A. (2014). Towards prescribed music in clinical contexts: More than words. *Music and Medicine, 6*(2), 70–77.

Royal Conservatory of Music. (2014). *The benefits of music education.* Toronto, Ontario, Canada: Author.

Ruud, E. (2010). *Music therapy: A perspective from the humanities.* Gilsum, NH: Barcelona.

Saxe, G. N., Ellis, B. H., & Brown, A. D. (2015). *Trauma systems therapy for children and teens.* New York: Guilford Publications.

Saarikallio, S., & Erkkilä, J. (2007). The role of music in adolescents' mood regulation. *Psychology of Music, 35*(1), 88–109.

Salimpoor, V. N., Benovoy, M., Larcher, K., Dagher, A., & Zatorre, R. J. (2011). Anatomically distinct dopamine release during anticipation and experience of peak emotion to music. *Nature Neuroscience, 14*(2), 257–262.

Scaer, R. (2014). *The body bears the burden: Trauma, dissociation, and disease.* New York: Routledge.

Schellenberg, E. G. (2005). Music and cognitive abilities. *Current Directions in Psychological Science, 14*(6), 317–320.

Schlez, A., Litmanovitz, I., Bauer, S., Dolfin, T., Regev, R., & Arnon, S. (2011). Combining kangaroo care and live harp music therapy in the neonatal intensive care setting. *Israel Medical Association Journal, 13*(6), 354–358.

Schore, A. N. (2009). Relational trauma and the developing right brain: An interface of psychoanalytic self psychology and neuroscience. *Annals of the New York Academy of Sciences, 1159*(1), 189–203.

Schulz, C. (1967). *Happiness is a sad song.* San Francisco: Determined Productions.

Schwartz, E. (2008). *Music, therapy, and early childhood: A developmental approach.* Gilsum, NH: Barcelona.

Sears, W. W. (1968). Processes in music therapy. In E. T. Gaston (Ed.), *Music in therapy* (pp. 30–44). New York: Macmillan.

Seri, N., & Gilboa, A. (2017, March). When music therapists adopt an ethnographic approach: Discovering the music of ultra-religious boys in Israel. *Approaches: An Interdisciplinary Journal of Music Therapy, First View*, pp. 1–15.

Shahin, A. J., Roberts, L. E., Chau, W., Trainor, L. J., & Miller, L. M. (2008). Music training leads to the development of timbre-specific gamma band activity. *NeuroImage, 41*(1), 113–122.

Sherrod, K., Vietze, P., & Friedman, S. (1978). *Infancy.* Monterey, CA: Brooks/Cole.

Shiller, V. M. (2017). *The attachment bond: Affectional ties across the lifespan.* New York: Lexington Books.

Siegel, D. J. (2006). An interpersonal neurobiology approach to psychotherapy: Awareness, mirror neurons, and neural plasticity in the development of well-being. *Psychiatric Annals, 36*(4), 248–256.

Siegel, D. J. (2012). *The developing mind: How relationships and the brain interact to shape who we are* (2nd ed.). New York: Guilford Press.

Skoe, E., & Kraus, N. (2012). A little goes a long way : How the adult brain is shaped by musical training in childhood. *Journal of Neuroscience, 32*(34), 11507–11510.

Small, C. (1998). *Musicking.* Middletown, CT: Wesleyan University Press.

Smart, M. S., & Smart, R. C. (1978). *Infants: Development and relationships* (2nd ed.). New York: Macmillan.

Soke, G. N., Rosenberg, S. A., Hamman, R. F., Fingerlin, T., Robinson, C., Carpenter, L., . . . DiGuiseppe, C. (2016). Brief report: Prevalence of self-injurious behaviors among children with autism spectrum disorder—a population-based study. *Journal of Autism and Developmental Disorders, 46*(11), 3607–3614.

Soley, G., & Spelke, E. S. (2016). Shared cultural knowledge: Effects of music on young children's social preferences. *Cognition, 148*, 106–116.

Standley, J. M. (2002). *Music techniques in therapy, counseling, and special education* (2nd ed.), St. Louis, MO: MMB Music.

Steele, P. H. (1984). Aspects of resistance in music therapy: Theory and technique. *Music Therapy, 4*(1), 64–72.

Stern, D. N. (1985). *The interpersonal world of the infant*. New York: Basic Books.
Stern, D. N. (2008). The clinical relevance of infancy: A progress report. *Infant Mental Health Journal, 29*(3), 177–188.
Stern, D. N. (2010). *Forms of vitality: Exploring dynamic experience in psychology, the arts, psychotherapy and development*. Oxford, UK: Oxford University Press.
Stewart, A. L., Field, T. A., & Echterling, L. G. (2016). Neuroscience and the magic of play. *International Journal of Play Therapy, 25*(1), 4–13.
Stewart, A. L., Whelan, W. F., & Pendleton, C. (2014). Attachment theory as a road map for play therapists. In C. A. Malchiodi & D. A. Crenshaw (Eds.), *Creative arts and play therapy for attachment problems* (pp. 25–51). New York: Guilford Press.
Stewart, K. (Ed.). (2010). *Music therapy and trauma: Bridging theory and clinical practice*. New York: Satchnote Press.
Stormshak, E. A., DeVargas, E., & Cárdenas, L. E. (2017). Parenting practices and the development of problem behavior. In J. E. Lochman & W. Matthys (Eds.), *The Wiley handbook of disruptive and impulse-control disorders* (pp. 307–322). Chichester, UK: Wiley.
Storr, A. (1991). Music in relation to the self. *Journal of British Music Therapy, 5*(1), 5–13.
Suzuki, S. (1969). *Nurtured by love: A new approach to education* (W. Suzuki, Trans.). New York: Exposition Press.
Swain, J., Hancock, K., Dixon, A., Koo, S., & Bowman, J. (2013). Acceptance and commitment therapy for anxious children and adolescents: Study protocol for a randomized controlled trial. *Trials, 14*(1), 140.
Taylor, D. (2010). *Biomedical foundations of music as therapy* (2nd ed.). Eau Claire, WI: Barton.
Temporal Dynamics of Learning Center. (n.d.). Music and the brain. Retrieved from *http://tdlc.ucsd.edu/research/highlights/rh-music-and-brain-2011.html*.
Thompson, R. A. (2016). Early attachment and later development: Reframing the questions. In J. Cassidy & P. R. Shaver (Eds.), *Handbook of attachment: Theory, research, and clinical applications* (3rd ed., pp. 330–348). New York: Guilford Press.
Thompson, W. F., Schellenberg, E. G., & Husain, G. (2004). Decoding speech prosody: Do music lessons help? *Emotion, 4*(1), 46–64.
Trainor, L., Shahin, A., & Roberts, L. (2003). Effects of musical training on the auditory cortex in children. *Annals of the New York Academy of Sciences, 999*(1), 506–513.
Trevarthen, C. (1994). The self born in intersubjectivity: The psychology of an infant communicating. In U. Neisser (Ed.), *The perceived self: Ecological and interpersonal sources of self knowledge* (pp. 121–173). New York: Cambridge University Press.

Trevarthen, C. (1997). Preface. In M. Pavlicevic, *Music therapy in context: Music, meaning and relationship* (pp. ix–xii). London: Jessica Kingsley.

Trevarthen, C. (2002). Origins of musical identity: Evidence from infancy for musical social awareness. In R. A. R. MacDonald, D. J. Hargreaves, & D. Miell (Eds.), *Musical identities* (pp. 21–38). Oxford, UK: Oxford University Press.

Trevarthen, C., Aitken, K., Papoudi, D., & Robarts, J. (1998). *Children with autism*. London: Jessica Kingsley.

Trevarthen, C., & Malloch, S. N. (2000). The dance of wellbeing: Defining the musical therapeutic effect. *Nordic Journal of Music Therapy, 9*(2), 3–17.

Trevarthen, C., & Panksepp, J. (2017). In tune with feeling: Musical play with emotions of creativity, inspiring neuroaffective development and self-confidence for learning in company. In S. Hart (Ed.), *Inclusion, play and empathy: Neuroaffective development in children's groups* (pp. 29–54). Philadelphia: Jessica Kingsley.

Trondalen, G., & Skarderud, F. (2007). Playing with affects. *Nordic Journal of Music Therapy, 16*(2), 100–111.

Tronick, E. (2007). *The neurobehavioral and social emotional development of infants and children*. New York: Norton.

Trost, W., Labbé, C., & Grandjean, D. (2017). Rhythmic entrainment as a musical affect induction mechanism. *Neuropsychologia, 96*, 96–110.

Tsang, C. D., Falk, S., & Hessel, A. (2017). Infants prefer infant-directed song over speech. *Child Development, 88*(4), 1207–1215.

Turry, A. (2002). Don't let the fear prevent the grief: Working with traumatic reactions through improvisation. In J. V. Loewy & A. F. Hara (Eds.), *Caring for the caregiver: The use of music and music therapy in grief and trauma* (pp. 44–53). Silver Springs, MD: American Music Therapy Association.

Upadhyay, D. K., Shukla, R., Tripathi, V. N., & Agrawal, M. (2017). Exploring the nature of music engagement and its relation to personality among young adults. *International Journal of Adolescence and Youth, 22*(4), 1–13.

Van den Tol, A. J. M., & Edwards, J. (2013). Exploring a rationale for choosing to listen to sad music when feeling sad. *Psychology of Music, 41*(4), 440–465.

van der Kolk, B. A. (2006). Clinical implications of neuroscience research in PTSD. *Annals of the New York Academy of Sciences, 1071*(1), 277–293.

van der Kolk, B. A. (2017). Developmental trauma disorder: Toward a rational diagnosis for children with complex trauma histories. *Psychiatric Annals, 35*(5), 401–408.

van der Kolk, B. A., Roth, S., Pelcovitz, D., Sunday, S., & Spinazzola, J. (2005). Disorders of extreme stress: The empirical foundation of a complex adaptation to trauma. *Journal of Traumatic Stress, 18*(5), 389–399.

VanFleet, R., & Faa-Thompson, T. (2017). Animal assisted play therapy with reticent children. In C. A. Malchiodi & D. A. Crenshaw (Eds.), *What to do* when children clam up in psychotherapy (pp. 217–237). New York: Guilford Press.

Varèse, E., & Wen-Chung, C. (1966). The liberation of sound. *Perspectives of New Music, 5*(1), 11–19.

Vuoskoski, J. K., & Eerola, T. (2017). The pleasure evoked by sad music is mediated by feelings of being moved. *Frontiers in Psychology, 8*, article 439.

Vuoskoski, J. K., Thompson, W. F., McIlwain, D., & Eerola, T. (2012). Who enjoys listening to sad music and why? *Music Perception: An Interdisciplinary Journal, 29*(3), 311–317.

Winner, E., Goldstein, T., & Vincent-Lancrin, S. (2013). *Art for art's sake?: The impact of arts education.* Paris: OECD.

Winnicott, D. W. (1971). *Playing and reality.* New York: Tavistock.

Winston, F. K., Kassam-Adams, N., Garcia-España, F., Ittenbach, R., & Cnaan, A. (2003). Screening for risk of persistent posttraumatic stress in injured children and their parents. *JAMA, 290*(5), 643–649.

Wittkowski, A., Cartwright, K., Emsley, R., Bee, P., Calam, R., Cross, C., . . . Reid, H. (2018). Enhancing maternal and infant wellbeing: study protocol for a feasibility trial of the Baby Triple P Positive Parenting programme for mothers with severe mental health difficulties (the IMAGINE study). *Trials, 19*(1), 479.

Young, L. N., Cordes, S., & Winner, E. (2013). Arts involvement predicts academic achievement only when the child has a musical instrument. *Educational Psychology, 34*(7), 849–861.

Zanetti, C. A., Powell, B., Cooper, G., & Hoffman, K. (2011). The Circle of Security intervention: Using the therapeutic relationship to ameliorate attachment security in disorganized dyads. In J. Solomon & C. George (Eds.), *Disorganized attachment and caregiving* (pp. 318–342). New York: Guilford Press.

Zeifman, D. M., & Hazan, C. (2016). Pair bonds as attachments: Mounting evidence in support of Bowlby's hypothesis: Attachment and psychopathology in childhood. In J. Cassidy & P. R. Shaver (Eds.), *Handbook of attachment: Theory, research, and clinical applications* (3rd ed., pp. 416–434). New York: Guilford Press.

Zilberstein, K. (2014). The use and limitations of attachment theory in child psychotherapy. *Psychotherapy, 51*(1), 93–103.

Zubala, A., & Karkou, V. (2015). Dance movement psychotherapy practice in the UK. *Body, Movement and Dance in Psychotherapy, 10*(1), 21–38.

Index

The letter *f* following a page number indicates figure; the letter *t* indicates table.

"ABC Song," 12, 34, 104, 114, 163
Adolescents.
 music impacts and, 141
 musical responsiveness and, 96–97
Affirmation, music as, 70–71
American Music Therapy Association, 4
Anxiety disorder, vignette, 164–165
Attachment
 disrupted, 107–108
 theories of, 107–109
Attachment problems
 group work and, 127–129
 practice recommendations, 129–130
 working with, 115–120
 vignettes, 116–120
Attachment-based interventions, 107–109
 with parents/caregivers, 121–126
Attention, music training and, 84–85
Attention-deficit/hyperactivity disorder (ADHD), prevalence of, 157
Attunement
 music and, 113–114
 process of, 111–114
 vignette, 122–123
Autism spectrum disorder (ASD)
 attunement and, 114
 and experience of time, 9–10
 impairments in, 169
 interventions in, 169–171
 prevalence of, 157
 routines and, 167
 sound sensitivity and, 31
 vignettes, 171–173

B

Behavior, prosocial
 encouraging, 161–162
 vignette, 162–163
Behavioral, emotional, and communication disorders, 157–176
 music as supportive intervention, 158–169
 for children with ASD, 169–172
 for creating routines/facilitating transitions, 167–169
 for encouraging prosocial behavior, 161–163
 for facilitating language, 159–160
 for identifying emotions, 165–166
 for organized communication/ interactions, 160–161
 practice recommendations, 173–176
 for regulating high levels of emotion, 163–165
 nonmusical interventions for, 158
Behaviors, disorganized, 160
 vignette, 161
Bells, 51
Bereavement; *see* Grief/bereavement

Index

Biases, letting go of, 63–65
Body parts, songs about, 34
Brain; *see also* Neuroscience
   music and language areas of, 83–84
   and response to trauma, 134
Breathing techniques, benefits of, 126, 131
Briggs's phases of musical development, 90–92
Bullying, musical dramas and, 46

C

Catharsis, moving beyond, 140
Change, music as agent of; *see* Music as agent of change
Chants, creating, 45, 48, 49, 76–77, 92, 136–137
Child(ren), musical history/preferences of, 57–58
Child abuse, vignette, 145–147
Child development, typical, 80–83
Child development and music
   in adolescence, 1–2, 81–83, 96–97
   culture and, 99
   emotions and, 98–99
   group work and, 104–105
   music participation and, 86, 87t, 88–90
   musical development and, 90–93, 94t–96t
   neuroscience of, 83–86
   practice recommendations, 102–104
   vignette, 99–102
Circle of Security (COS) intervention, 108–109, 121
Cognition, music and, 82, 87t
Cognitive abilities, increasing, 21
Communication
   disorganized, vignette, 161
   music as, 2–3, 113–114
   between newborns and mothers, 121
   nonverbal, 1
   psychobiological aspects of, 108
Communication disorders; *see* Behavioral, emotional, and communication disorders
Conduct disorder (CD)
   facial expression identification and, 165
   prevalence of, 157
   vignette, 166
Control; *see* Sense of control
Creative (now) time, 8
Creativity, music and, 83

Cultural influences
   grief and, 100–102
   musical development and, 99
   vignette, 99–102
   and working with parents, 124–125

D

Dance, music and, 61–62
Dance/movement therapy (DMT), 61–62
Dialectical behavior therapy (DBT), 143
Disorganized communication/behavior, 160–161
Disruptive behaviors, functions of, 72
Dissociation, posttraumatic, 144–147
   vignette, 145–147
Dissonance
   musical, 71
   trauma and, 133
Dopamine, music and release of, 2
Down syndrome, vignette, 161
Dramas
   mini-musical, 103
   musical, 46
Drumming, 24–25, 37–38
   attachment problems and, 115
   as communication, 5
   following trauma, 136–137
   "goodbye effect" and, 177–178
   for identifying emotions, 155
Drums, 50–51, 53f
Dynamics, 15–16
   children's use of, 5

E

Early Start Denver Model, 169
Einstein, Albert, 81
Elementary school children, musical development in, 96t
Emotional disorders; *see* Behavioral, emotional, and communication disorders
Emotion regulation
   after trauma, 142–144
   in behavioral, emotional, and communication disorders, 163–165
   vignette, 164–165

music and, 71–73
therapist guidelines, 77
Emotional time, 8
Emotions
  identifying, 165
    vignette, 166
  music and, 98–99
  sounding, 155–156
"Emotions game," 130
Entrainment, process of, 110–111
Executive functions, music training and, 84–85

F

"Fair Katrinelje and Pif-Paf-Poltrie," 128–129
Feedback, useful, 66–69
Feelings, musical reflection of, 62
Flow of time
  child's experience of, 6–7
  music and, 7

G

Gaston, E. Thayer, 4
Glockenspiel, 51
Goals, 20–21
"Goodbye effect," 177
Grief/bereavement, 147–150
  cultural influences on, 100–102
  vignettes, 148–150
Group work with music, 45–46
  child development and, 104–105
  musical development and, 104–105
  prosocial behavior and, 161–163
  recommendations for, 49
  for relationship problems, 127–129
  turn taking and, 174–175
Growth time, 7
Guiros, 23f

H

Haek, John, 13
Harmony, consonant *versus* dissonant, 14–15
Headphones, noise-cancelling, 31
Hearing, fetal development of, 80
"Home on the Range," 153

I

Imagery, working with, 43–45
Improvisation, 39–41
  for identifying emotions, 156
  in trauma therapy, 156
Impulse control, and working with music form/structure, 42–43
Impulse-control problems, vignette, 162–163
Infants/toddlers, musical development in, 80–81, 94t–95t
Instrumental music, listening to, 31–32
Instruments; *see* Musical instruments
Interpersonal relationships, 106–131
  at-risk children and, 106
  attachment and, 106–107 (*see also* Attachment; Attachment problems)
  attunement and, 111–114
    music and, 113–114
    vignette, 122–123
  entrainment and, 110–111
  group work and, 127–129
  parents/caregivers and, 121–126
    NICU and, 123–126
    vignette, 122–123
  polyvagal theory and, 109–110
  practice recommendations, 129–130
Interventions, attachment-based, 107–109, 121–126

K

Karaoke, 151

L

Language delays, working with, 33–34
Language development, music and, 82–83, 87t
Language production/comprehension, music in facilitation of, 159–160
Listening to music together, 31–32, 62–63, 148–149, 151, 174
Lullabies, 80, 131
  characteristics of, 3
  in NICU, 126
  routines and, 168
Lyrics; *see* Song lyrics

M

Melody, 11–12
Memory, music training and, 84–85
Metallophone, 24–26, 51
Mirror neurons, 110–111
Movement, music and, 33, 61–62
Music
    benefits of, 87t
    child development and (see Child development and music)
    children's responses to, 11
    choosing, 38
    components of, 10–17, 68–69
        dynamics, 15–16
        form, 16–17
        harmony, 14–15
        melody, 11–12
        rhythm, 13
        timbre, 13–14
    cultural expectations for, 2–3
    neuroscience findings and, 2, 83–86
    polyvagal theory and, 110
    speech/language centers and, 103
    talking about, 65–66
    time in (see Time experience)
    Web applications for, 38
Music as agent of change
    affirmations and, 70–71
    with different therapeutic approaches, 58–62
    emotion regulation and, 71–73
    and letting go of biases, preferences, 63–65
    and listening, being present, 62–63
    practice recommendations, 76–78
    resistance in therapy and, 73–75
    and talking about music, 65–66
    therapeutic skills and, 62
    vignettes, 66–70, 75–76
Music in Therapy (Gaston), 4
Music making, participation in, 86, 88–90
Music therapy, 3–6
    benefits of, 22–26
    children's responses to, 4–5, 23
    choice of instrument and, 14
    cotreating in, 27
    getting started activities, 29–56
        improvisation, 39–41
        instrument/equipment recommendations, 50–52, 53f–56f
        introducing instruments, 37–38
        listening to instrumental music/songs, 31–32
        music in group work, 45–46
        music-friendly office set-up, 29–31
        singing confidence and, 32–33
        vignette, 35–37
        working with imagery and themes, 43–45
        working with lyrics, 33–35
        working with music form and structure, 42–43
    goals in, 20–22
    negative potential of, 138–140
    origins of, 3–4
    personal preferences and, 18–19
    practice recommendations, 47–49
        for client groups, 49
        for individual clients, 47–49
    as psychological first aid, 140–141
    recommendations for practice, 27–28
    therapist confidence and, 17–18
    using, 17–19
Music Together, 93
Musical development
    benefits of, 81–83
    Briggs's phases of, 90–92
    in fetus/infant, 80–81
    models of, 90–93, 94t–96t
    Schwartz's response levels and, 92–93
Musical form/structure, 16–17, 42–43
Musical instruments, 53f–56f
    exploring, 154–155
    improvisation with, 40
    selection recommendations, 50–52
    timbre of, 14
    in trauma therapy, 154–155
    using, 37–38
Musical intervals, 12
Musical patterns, timbre and, 14
Musical preferences
    of child, 57–58
    of therapist, 63–65
Musical training, impacts on brain, 84–85
Musicking, 86, 88
"My Favorite Things," 153

N

"Name Game," 175
National Association for Music Therapy, 4